FITNESS AFTER 40

Second Edition

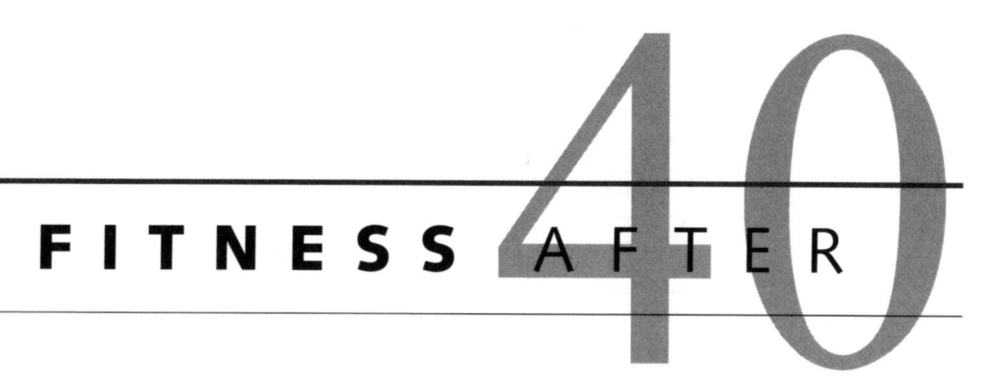

YOUR STRONG BODY AT 40, 50, 60, AND BEYOND

Includes a 6-Week Total-Body Workout Program

Vonda Wright, M.D., M.S.
Director of PRIMA™
(Performance and Research Initiative for Masters Athletes),
UPMC Center for Sports Medicine;
and Medical Director,
UPMC Lemieux Sports Complex

WITH *Ruth Winter, M.S.*

AMACOM

AMERICAN MANAGEMENT ASSOCIATION

New York • Atlanta • Brussels • Chicago • Mexico City • San Francisco
Shanghai • Tokyo • Toronto • Washington, D.C.

Bulk discounts available. For details visit:
www.amacombooks.org/go/specialsales
Or contact special sales:
Phone: 800–250–5308
Email: specialsls@amanet.org
View all the AMACOM titles at: www.amacombooks.org
American Management Association: www.amanet.org

Photos 1–5 are used with permission of Dr. Vonda Wright's Guide to Thrive: Four Steps to Body, Brains, and Bliss *(Chicago, Ill.: Triumph Books, 2011).*

Library of Congress Cataloging-in-Publication Data

Wright, Vonda.
Fitness after 40 : your strong body at 40, 50, 60, and beyond / Vonda Wright, M.D., with Ruth Winter.
pages cm
Includes bibliographical references and index.
ISBN 978-0-8144-4900-4 (pbk.) — ISBN 0-8144-4900-X (pbk.) — ISBN 978-0-8144-4902-8 (ebook) — ISBN 0-8144-4902-6 (ebook) 1. Exercise for middle-aged persons. 2. Physical fitness for middle-aged persons. 3. Middle-aged persons—Health and hygiene. I. Winter, Ruth, 1930– II. Title.

GV482.6.W75 2015
613.7'044—dc23

2014046996

About AMA
American Management Association (www.amanet.org) is a world leader in talent development, advancing the skills of individuals to drive business success. Our mission is to support the goals of individuals and organizations through a complete range of products and services, including classroom and virtual seminars, webcasts, webinars, podcasts, conferences, corporate and government solutions, business books, and research. AMA's approach to improving performance combines experiential learning—learning through doing—with opportunities for ongoing professional growth at every step of one's career journey.

Printing number
10 9 8 7 6 5 4 3 2 1

Caring for masters athletes, whether they are winning races or stepping back into a life of mobility, is a true joy and inspiration. I am forever grateful for their persistence in life and for helping me dispel the myth that aging is an inevitable decline from vitality to frailty! Masters athletes prove we can be healthy, vital, active, and joyful at every age and skill level.

LOVE, and all my best, to my husband, **PETER**; our blended family of six who are keeping us young, **PAT**, **JOHN**, **ANDREW**, **LOUIS**, **COREY**, and **ISABELLA**; and my ever-youthful parents, **GENE** and **JOY**.

—Dr. Vonda

CONTENTS

ACKNOWLEDGMENTS

The growth of *Fitness After 40,* from merely an inspiration to the force igniting a national platform for changing the way we age in this country, has been an incredible journey for me and the thousands of athletes, adult-onset exercisers, and once-upon-a-timers who have taken control of our aging process and believe that the best days of our lives are now!

When I wrote the first edition of *Fitness After 40*, I had to convince people that 40 and beyond were not just birthdays mourned with black balloons and sad farewells to youth. Now I am overjoyed that crowds of people agree with me that 40 and older is not just a "cool" age but can actually be the prime of our lives. As I step back to appraise the last six years since *Fitness After 40* first ignited a national conversation on active aging, I realize that I have many contributors to whom I am very grateful.

Of course, I must thank God and my family. God for giving me a mind capable of invention, and the hands and drive to make it happen. My parents, Gene and Joy Wright, who raised me to believe that anything I wanted to do was possible. My husband, Peter Taglianetti, for being a solid rock of support as I follow my passions. I am most thankful for my precious blessing,

Isabella, who is smart, sweet, and adventurous and motivates everything I do now.

I thank Ruth Winter, my coauthor, for her experience that guided me through the literary forest, one that is so different from medicine. Ruth would like to thank her late husband, Arthur Winter, M.D., for his support. I thank Ruth for introducing me to Linda Konner, our fabulous literary agent, who courageously championed our original proposal to publishers and continues to skillfully guide me through the process, embracing my vision even when I push. Like a surgeon, she is both tough and compassionate; I like that.

I thank Amacom for bringing *Fitness After 40* out of my office and to the world. Specifically, I thank Robert Nirkind, our editor, for giving my vision renewed life and for being the cohesive force that combined all the elements of this book. I am thankful to the Amacom team: Michael Sivilli, our associate editor, for expertly managing the details of the manuscript preparation; Irene Majuk, for charging forth with PR; Jacqueline Laks Gorman and Alison Hagge, for their hard work in envisioning how this book should be presented visually; and the army of behind-the-scenes people at Amacom, whom I never had the privilege to meet, but who worked diligently on this book.

Special thanks to Chad Biddinger, masters sprint tri-athlete, and Laura Petrilla, our photographer (misslphotography.com).

Studying Senior Olympians and maturing athletes is both fascinating and inspiring. I am thankful to the National Senior Games Association for allowing me access to their remarkable athletes during the 2001 and 2005 games, and to the more than 3,000 senior athletes who participated in our studies. Also, I cannot forget the guidance of Peter Z. Cohen, M.D., who first turned me on to the Senior Olympics, and Robin Waxenberg, who built the media and PR base for *Fitness After 40*.

Finally, I must thank my chairman, Dr. Freddie H. Fu, and my colleagues at the UPMC Center for Sports Medicine who helped me turn my vision for a Performance and Research Initiative for Masters Athletes (PRIMA) into a thriving venue for maturing athletes of all skill levels. Through our PRIMA programs, PRIMA Start and PRIMA Athlete, we assist these remarkable people to raise their performances to the next level while minimizing injury.

Fitness After 40 captures the conversations I have with my patients daily. My patients inspire me to keep thinking of new ideas and to always strive to be a better surgeon. It is a privilege to be their doctor.

—Vonda Wright, M.D.

"Go confidently in the direction of your dreams. Live the life you have imagined."

—Henry David Thoreau, American author, poet, and philosopher

INTRODUCTION

My vision is to change the way we age in this country. There is a myth out there that aging involves an inevitable decline from the vitality of youth to the frailty of old age. This simply is not true. *You* have the power to dispel that myth in your own life.

You control more than 70 percent of your health and aging process by the decisions *you* make *today*. Only 30 percent of how you age is determined by your genetics (so it's time to stop blaming your parents). *You* are in the driver's seat and *you* control both today and much of your future.

The first edition of *Fitness After 40: How to Stay Strong at Any Age* helped ignite a national conversation on active aging and empowered you—in the best half of your life—to take control of your body and master how it ages. At the time of its launch, interest in this topic was in its infancy and the book brought the topic into focus. In fact, it served as the nationwide foundation to explain and urge active aging. *Fitness After 40* empowered thousands of active agers and masters athletes alike. They, in turn, have participated in multiple community and corporate fitness programs based on the book during the last five years.

The second edition of *Fitness After 40* now capitalizes on the foundation laid by the original book and completely updates the content in line with current science and mobility trends. One of the joys of writing a second edition of *Fitness After 40* is sharing with you the amazing stories of my patients and friends who took control of their health, lost weight, and won new races. They now not only look healthier but feel stronger and are younger on the inside than they were five years ago.

As an orthopaedic surgeon and "mobility doc," I know that—no matter what your age or ability level—you were designed to move, and it is never too late to start.

Now is the time to maximize your performance and fitness, whether this means simply taking your first steps off the couch or ramping up to win your race age division. Your tools are mobility, smart nutrition, and believing that *you* are in control.

Here's what's new in this edition:

- The latest updates on the new "science of aging." We have discovered the fountain of youth!
- A decade-by-decade guide to maximizing your health, including tips about how building a better body also builds a stronger brain!
- Twenty-six brand new resistance exercises, detailed in step-by-step instructions and clearly illustrated, which (together, with the 15 resistance exercises from the first edition) systematically work your whole body.
- A series of 20 Minutes to Burn exercise "bricks." Each Burn circuit integrates five resistance exercises and creates a smart sequence that rigorously works one body area in 20 minutes.

- Quick-reference icons to mark the exercises that are designed to prevent or minimize the four most common injuries and causes of pain among athletes over 40.
- The new Six-Week Jump Start to Mobility Plan, which walks you, day by day, through an increasingly demanding workout schedule that systematically integrates the four components of F.A.C.E.-ing your fitness after 40 (through the components of Flexibility, Aerobic Exercise, Carry a Load, and Equilibrium/Balance).
- A specially designed section of "cheat sheets" for the nine 20 Minutes to Burn circuits. Each cheat sheet features quick visual and text references to the five resistance exercises that are included in the circuit. This section is designed so you can photocopy a page or snap a photo with a phone—and literally take the Fitness to Go concept (introduced in the first edition) to the next level.
- An overhauled nutrition chapter, which deals with smart nutrition based on real science to minimize the aches and pains of aging via building an anti-inflammatory environment in your body. In addition, discussions about macronutrients, micronutrients, supplements, and nutrition for vegetarian and vegan athletes have been vastly expanded since the last edition. What you eat determines how you feel!
- Four new chapters for making *Fitness After 40* the start of the best years of your life!

FITNESS AFTER 40

Second Edition

"Credit belongs to the man who is actually in the arena, whose face is marred by . . . sweat and blood; . . . who at the best knows in the end the triumph of high achievement, and who at the worst, if he fails, at least fails while daring greatly."

—President Theodore Roosevelt

CHAPTER ONE

1

You Are Strong, You Are Powerful, You Move You!

I love taking care of people. It is pure joy to lead a group of patients from the couch to a 5K race and see their entire perspective on their future change. Their bodies become stronger and fitter, but more importantly, their minds come to believe they can actively control their health with the decisions they make each day. And they are right!

A new generation of mature athletes and adult-onset exercisers (AOEs) are changing the very paradigm of aging. They are not satisfied with a superficial veneer of youth but are remaining youthful on the inside—as well as on the outside—through mobility. In fact, those who push themselves to the next level through competition are more mentally and physically healthy than their sedentary counterparts. Mature athletes and AOEs are a remarkable and growing group of people. They are not waiting for age to overtake them; they are proactively taking steps toward aging to perfection.

After 29 years of taking care of patients and athletes of every skill and age level, I have learned that no amount of education, hand-holding, or even public humiliation (as is commonly seen on TV) will motivate people to make real change in their lives and health. People make change only when *they* decide they are worth it, and then they move themselves.

You have heard me say it before—70 percent of your health and aging is controlled by the decisions you make today. *You* are a powerful force in your own future. Your decision to take control is not likely to happen because it is important to your spouse, your boss, your kids, or your friends. It will happen because *you* decide that you are important enough to invest the time daily in the decisions that will change your life. *You* are powerful. *You* are strong. *You* move *you*!

MARY BETH'S STORY

Mary Beth is the wife of my daughter's basketball coach. Every Sunday night for the last two years, she has shown up at practices to organize us, pitch in wherever and whenever she was needed, and generally run the show. She would tell you that—although she managed her family and work—at twice her healthy size, she was not at her best.

Last year, we showed up to begin the season and Mary Beth was different. In fact, I barely recognized her! She looked younger and infinitely more healthy. She had lost 100 pounds. Wow! I was *really* proud of Mary Beth. And at times like this, I am often seen jumping up and down and hugging someone. Mary Beth had dramatically taken control of her health and future.

When she shared her story with me, I was silent and humbled. After the previous basketball season, Mary Beth's husband had picked up a copy of *Fitness After 40* as a present for her. As she was reading it, something clicked inside her. She internalized my message that smart nutrition and mobility could change her life. She realized that she is important and that the small decisions she made *each day* were important. She could be strong. She could be powerful. She could move to her best health, and she did!

IN MARY BETH'S OWN WORDS

I looked at a picture from vacation and decided it was time to take care of myself and lose the weight I had gained over the years. I went to the doctor to have some blood tests done, and my numbers were extremely high. I decided right then that I had to make a change—and make it *that day*.

My husband, Tim, bought me *Fitness After 40* by Dr. Vonda Wright. I stopped drinking soda pop and eating fast food. I bought whole-wheat English muffins and a lot of raw vegetables. Water and milk were the only beverages I drank. I cut up vegetables and put them in containers so they were ready to eat when I got hungry. I had a game plan that I could live with.

I dusted off an old aerobics video that my husband had bought for me when we were dating, and I did the exercises six times a week for 40 minutes. Now, I get upset with myself if a day goes by and I don't get in my exercise. It used to be a chore, but exercising is so much fun now, and the results keep me excited about doing it as much as possible. Everyone has a half hour each day to give to themselves to exercise. My motto is: "No excuses!"

I lost 100 pounds in six months. I went from a size 20 to a size 4. I was 250 pounds, and now I am an exciting 144. My husband took me shopping, and I had so much fun trying on all new stuff. I feel so much better about myself! I no longer get out of breath walking up the steps in our house. Now I enjoy taking pictures with my husband and children, and I like the way that I look. I love keeping up with my exercise schedule and watching what I eat.

It is not a diet. It has become a lifestyle. I love walking into a room with my husband and children, looking good and knowing they are proud of me. Thank you for all your support, Tim, Kyle, and Angela. I love you all so much.

YOU ARE STRONG!

If you have picked up this book, you are at least thinking about what it means to be strong and powerful. No more huffing and puffing on the stairs; no more longing for energy. You want to feel vigorous and have the oomph to do the things you want, not to mention look strong in your clothes. Living this life starts on the inside and moves its way out. And the key is health through mobility.

I want you to understand—before you think I am simply another workout cheerleader in an orthopaedist's clothing—that I realize there can be real barriers on the road to healthy aging. I understand being busy, getting pulled in 20 directions at once, having family obligations, and dealing with financial constraints. I understand the dozens of other very logical (and some not so logical) reasons my patients offer up every day in my office. Here are some of the top excuses I've heard from my patients—and my replies:

- "I run around all day. Isn't that enough exercise?" *No! Your heart rate must be elevated for a minimum of 30 minutes a day.*
- "I can't afford to exercise." *Turn off your cable. Use the money to join a health club, and watch TV there.*
- "I think about it all the time, but I don't know where to begin." *Read this book and get up off the couch.*
- "We have a treadmill and an elliptical machine, but they are covered with clothes." *That is the most expensive clothes hanger I ever heard of. You know what to do.*
- "Even though I haven't exercised in 20 years, I used to be a Navy SEAL and do incredible physical feats. I can't bring myself to start exercising like a beginner." *After 20 years off, your body is like a beginner's. Let's go.*
- "The dog ate my sneakers . . . . "

When he'd run out of excuses for why he was still sitting on the couch, one of my patients actually told me that his dog *had* eaten his sneakers. He was one of my favorite patients, and he said it with a straight face. For an instant, I considered him seriously before a smirk settled in on his face and we both burst into laughter. He wanted to be one of those svelte older men who looked and felt younger than the age on his driver's license, yet he had not made a move to get there. The truth is that 78 percent of people over 50 years old cite exercise as the key to aging well, but only 28 percent are currently doing anything about it.

No matter what your excuse or excuses may be, the fact remains that unless you take the time to invest in active aging now, you will likely be forced to take the time to deal with illness in the future. Therefore, let's just put some of the major exercise barriers out on the table and hash them out. The three most common exercise barriers in my patients are "couch addiction," injury, and osteoarthritis.

BARRIERS TO EXERCISE

Couch addiction. Am I serious? Well, not entirely, and yet the habit of spending our lives as couch potatoes is a serious threat. I understand the issue—the lure of sinking into the soft sanctuary of the sofa after a hard day of work. In fact, during the beginning of my residency, I specifically bought my couch with napping in mind. At the local department store, I took flying leaps onto the laps of couch after couch, seeking the perfect place to take my naps. After a 36-hour "workday," my couch provided much-needed relief.

The problem is that too much of a good thing *can* kill you. According to some of our nation's top physiologists, physical inactivity is a serious health threat and will lead to premature disability or death in more than 2.5 million Americans in the next 10 years. Thirty-five common diseases are made worse when people are physically inactive, including diabetes, high blood pressure, heart disease, and stroke. In addition, women who spend two hours a day in front of the TV have a 23 percent greater chance of being obese compared to women who do not. I wish there was an easy way to tell you how to break the habit of spending hours every evening sitting on the couch, watching TV. You simply have to make a real commitment to "just do it!" (as the Nike advertisements say). If you are a hopeless TV addict, then outsmart the problem and make your living room a home gym.

Regarding other barriers to exercise, it is true that those of us over 40 who exercise, and even those who don't, face the increased challenge of injury and arthritis. The number of people suffering from these problems is exceeded only by the products on the market promoting pain relief. Yet these two real and troublesome barriers to active aging do not have to be barriers at all. My entire career is geared to teaching athletes and active agers over 40 to be smarter as they avoid being sidelined. I not only treat their current injuries but work with them to prevent future injury and move past the aches and pains of arthritis. I look forward, in the following chapters, to sharing some of the information I give to my aspiring masters athletes and inspiring patients. (The term "masters athletes" describes a broad category of amateurs who remain competitive after college and into their forties, fifties, and beyond. Their goals can include winning the whole race, winning their age divisions, or topping their personal bests.)

Fitness After 40, however, is not just about exercising: It is about awakening the champion—the winner—within you. It represents years of research (my own and that of others) that can mean the difference between simply letting the aging process master you as opposed to making your next 40 years the best yet. Many of the commonly accepted stereotypes of aging are simply the effects of a sedentary lifestyle, not about real aging at all! Getting older does not mean being worse. Yes, there are changes. The truth is that no matter how fit you were at 20, after 40 you are a new you. You are simply not the same person you once were. However, not only can you still feel the strength and vigor of youth, you can perform nearly as well—and perhaps even better—physically than you did 10 or even 20 years ago.

Based on my research with Senior Olympians and as director of PRIMA (Performance and Research Initiative for Masters Athletes) at the UPMC Center for Sports Medicine, your best may be yet to come. In the five years since *Fitness After 40* was first published, hundreds of adult-onset exercisers—formerly couch potatoes—completed one of our 12-week exercise programs aimed at helping them get off the couch and finish a 5K walk/run. In our twice-weekly sessions, they received much of the same information found in this book. They exercised together twice a week and individually two to three times per week. To our joy, they repeatedly recount the life-changing experience of rising above their expectations of finishing the 5K race and actually medaling in their age divisions. Talk about feeling vigorous! There is nothing like raising the bar of your personal best to make you feel alive. These AOEs, like you, had the benefit of the experience and wisdom that comes with age. By putting aside their past excuses for not exercising, they took control and got into great shape. Many of our AOEs have continued their lifestyle of mobility and have become true runners. They continue to move themselves to their best health.

THE GOOD NEWS AND THE BAD NEWS

There is good news and bad news when it comes to remaining or becoming active after the age of 40. The good news is that increasing numbers of people over 40 are seeking ways to remain youthful by exercising. A survey of baby boomers—those born between 1946 and 1964—conducted by ThermaCare, a company that sells a heat pack that becomes warm when applied to the skin, found:

- 40 percent were living healthier lives and were more physically fit than when they were in their twenties
- 67 percent felt 11 years younger than their chronological age
- 57 percent reported being more physically active than their parents were at their age
- 33 percent boasted that they could beat their children in at least one sport

The people surveyed were either beginning to exercise for the first time (that is, they were AOEs) or were continuing programs they were already doing (active agers and athletes).

The bad news is that as we age, our bodies change, and these changes mean we are more vulnerable to injury. Injury is the Number 1 reason why people stop being active and the Number 2 reason (after the common cold) why people go to the doctor. These same baby boomer survey participants revealed that:

- 67 percent suffer from muscle or joint pain weekly
- 73 percent say muscle and joint pain is a bigger annoyance than making sure they remain physically active
- 69 percent claim they were willing to work through their pain to remain active

You will find as you go through this book that I don't believe in the mantra "No pain—no gain." My objective is to help you maximize your exercise efforts by smarter training while preventing the injuries that not only cause pain but keep you out of the game. If you do get hurt, you will find tips in this book on how to recover actively and without making things worse.

TALES FROM TWO AGING MASTERS ATHLETES

Since I began to work with mature athletes and watch the National Summer Senior Games, also known as the Senior Olympics—a biennial competition of a cross-section of ordinary and elite senior athletes (50 years old and older) who compete in 19 different sports—it has been a privilege and inspiration to know athletes such as 78-year-old Cliff Eggink. Cliff is the original "Irongeezer." Irongeezers range from baby boomers to ultraseniors, some of whom are in their eighties and nineties. Far from being cranky couch potatoes, these people have a passion for physical activity and involvement in a healthy lifestyle. They have a dash of "iron" for strength of mind and body to maintain hale and hardy lifestyles amid an increasingly slothful, unfit population.

"At 61 years," Cliff says, "I started trying to be healthy. I stayed off the medication and got out of the couch potato syndrome. Then everything just evolved. I had to push myself." Cliff did push himself. In 2005, at age 68, he was the oldest participant in the Ironman Arizona Triathlon competition. An Ironman Triathlon is 2.4 miles of swimming, followed by 112 miles of biking, followed by 26.2 miles of running. Cliff is inspiring as a competitive athlete, but so is my father, who just wants to be the best he can be for his physical and emotional health.

My father, Gene Wright, a former high school principal and entrepreneur and now a personal trainer, says:

> I made a decision early in my life to always be physically functional, emotionally stable, and personally happy. I did not want to be limited physically. Most of the adults that I knew could not move easily, abused themselves by their lifestyle choices, aged quickly, and developed the "aging

mobility syndrome." Most were unhealthy and had a long duration of physical dependence before they died.

I love life and living. I want to enjoy it for as long as I can. To me this seems worth working for. I am committed to being mobile. Throughout my life I have always been active and enjoyed running. I greatly enjoy running races. I enjoy the experience associated with them: the people, the places, and the things involved. I have participated in 5Ks, 10Ks, half marathons, and marathons. I still run and enjoy it.

During my 60 years of running, I have noticed some changes. My running efficiency declined from smooth, fluid, and flowing to labored and halting. My stride shortened and my pace went from six to 10 minutes per mile. My enjoyment while running (on a scale of 1 to 10) went from 8–9-10 to 3–4-5. It became hard and unpleasant to run. It became impossible to set another PR [personal record] at any distance.

At age 65, I sort of woke up and said, "Hey, fellow, if you want to run, things have to change." I needed an overhaul. I needed to rework my thinking, my conditioning routine, and my goals. In the years since, I have made both physical and mental changes. These were neither instantaneous nor easy.

Up until age 65 or so, the only conditioning program I had was to run every day, as hard as possible. I ran between 30 and 60 miles a week, every week. I raced (any distance—from a 5K to a half marathon) probably every other week. My motto was: "Get your shoes on, and hit the road, Jack, and don't look back." It was "go baby go," "don't miss a day," and "miles, miles, miles." My complete workout was devoted to running. During this period, I noticed that I was injured more and more and running less and less and frequently hitting the doldrums. It took longer and longer to recover.

This idea that I had to train harder, more intensely, and continually did not work. While I had been doing this for 40 years, it was no longer an effective strategy. It actually tore me apart. I needed to train differently. I needed to be smarter about my training.

At the age of 65, my training routine started to change. It became very different from my training when I was 40, 50, and 60. I started exercising five or six days a week with much variation and planned rest days. I realized that running is a total body activity and the total body needs to be trained. For almost 10 years, from age 65 on, my workout routine was varied and deliberate. I conditioned the total body. Running became only part of my weekly routine, even though it is still my favorite activity.

I embraced Vonda's "total body fitness" and "training smarter" philosophies she described in the first edition of *Fitness After 40*. We spend a lot of time working together to teach this method to thousands of active agers and adult-onset exercisers in Pittsburgh.

During this 10-year stretch, I started each workout with at least 10 minutes of total body dynamic warm-up. This was fun and prepared me for the rest of my workout. I followed this warm-up with a three- or four-mile walk/jog/run as many as four days a week. On some days I followed the warm-up with cross-training. Some days I ran and cross-trained; other days I cross-trained only. I did circuits of dynamic stretching/strength building, core training, cycling, swimming, and other activities. I also incorporated one day of complete rest each week. If I felt the need, I added another day of rest. I ended each workout with at least 10 minutes of cool-down time. This included walking, Static Stretching, and foam rolling. I found that this workout routine improved my mobility and my enjoyment while working out. I called this routine "working out smarter."

My physical approach to conditioning had changed. This was hard to accomplish. Old habits are not easy to change. My mindset is competitive. I love to win. If I can beat you to the finish line, *I will do it*. I still want to win my age group. I also knew that to qualify for the Boston Marathon, men 70 to 74 years old needed to run a marathon in 4:30.

Just when I felt as though I had found a new, workable, and smart system, my conditioning routine and running hit a big bump and came to a stop. For some unknown reason, avascular necrosis destroyed my left hip. I could not walk without great discomfort. Jogging was out of the question. There went any enjoyment I had from being mobile.

And then, on June 5, 2013, at the age of 73, I had a total hip replacement. I was "healed with steel." Fortunately, I had a great outcome: No hip joint pain, restored range of motion, and fluid mobility.

Two months after my surgery, I "ran" the Liberty Mile in Pittsburgh. A month later, I "ran" the Great Race 5K Run, also in Pittsburgh. I completed both races. Oh, yes, my Liberty Mile time was 15 minutes plus, and my Great Race 5K time was 47 minutes. But I finished both. What a great feeling!

Now, after rehab and a year of hard work, I can jog three to four miles comfortably. I am back on the road! Pretty good, I'd say. The mental change is as drastic as the physical change. My per-mile pace is now 13:30. But my time no longer matters to me, nor does my place of finish. What matters is that my friend—elation—is back, in everything I do: a workout, a cross-training, a run, a race. Elation. My friend is back! I am in shape, conditioned, and mobile. I have at least one success each day.

> It is greatly satisfying—to be mobile, to enjoy living. I wonder what is possible. Can I run a 5K, a 10K, 10 miles, a half marathon, a marathon? Can I stay vibrant, active, and happy through my seventies, eighties, nineties, and even hundreds? Can I enjoy family, community, and physical activity? Will living remain exciting and fulfilling?
>
> The answer is "yes." Mobility is great. Being healthy is great. Being happy is great. Bring on life!

Cliff and Gene don't need to be the exceptions. They can be the rule for maintaining strength and improving performance through exercise. Today's mature athletes and adult-onset exercisers have the potential to change the face and perception of aging in the United States. They are not bound to elderly behaviors in the same way their parents were. Today's athletes are unique; they are not merely sequels to their 20-year-old selves. They are highly active and motivated to stay young.

THIS IS ALL ABOUT YOU

Orthopaedic surgeons and other sports medicine professionals have done a tremendous job taking care of adolescent athletes, college athletes, and professional athletes. We have, however, virtually ignored the growing number of elite masters athletes and senior athletes over 40 years old who continue to remain active and fit.

I work with and study mature athletes and see their thrill when they are victorious in competition and their indomitable spirit when they are not. As I learned more about this dynamic group of people, I found that they have different needs from their younger counterparts. If you are over 40, for example, you need to train differently. This is because, although in your mind you still feel 25 years old, your body responds and recovers from injury differently than it did decades ago. Being more mature is actually an advantage in some endurance sports, such as running and swimming, but being smarter about beginning or increasing exercise and training is crucial. Adult-onset exercisers and masters athletes alike also have an advantage over their younger counterparts, as they are generally finished with their educations and, therefore, often have more control over their time and resources. These advantages, coupled with your desire to be the best you can be at every age, make the second half of your active life an exciting place to be. *The fact is that a 75-year-old athlete may still perform many times faster and be in better health than a sedentary 30- or 40-year-old.*

I believe there is no one-size-fits-all exercise program. Your exercise regime should be individualized for you, based on sound principles, and incorporated into your current activity. This book will help you recognize the capacity of your own body, adapt the principles described, and develop a fitness routine that fits within your lifestyle and abilities.

You can do more than you think you can. You can be stronger and more fit when you use the techniques described in this book. It will take determination and work, but as you travel through these pages, you will hear the same words I say every day to my patients. I hope you will feel like I am right there with you, helping you achieve your goals.

THE *FITNESS AFTER 40* Promise

If you are an elite masters athlete more than 40 years old, I can help you improve your performance. If you are a recreational athlete, I can encourage you to be your best and avoid injuries. If you are a couch potato, I can show you what you need to do to become fit. Let me tell you how you are going to achieve your goal.

In Chapter 2, you will learn exactly how your body becomes unique after you reach 40. You will be fascinated by the most recent studies showing the amazing effects of active aging and how you really do control 70 percent of your health.

In Chapter 3, you will discover the unique health and mobility issues for each decade of your life, and what you should do in that decade to maximize your current (and future!) health.

In Chapter 4, you will build a better brain as you learn about the profound and exciting connection between physical strength and fitness and how your brain and happiness can reap the benefits.

In Chapters 5, 6, 7, 8, and 9, you will learn how to F.A.C.E. your future. (F.A.C.E. is an acronym I use to help my patients remember the four components of fitness after 40 that you must include in your daily regimen: Flexibility, Aerobic Exercise, Carry a Load, and Equilibrium/Balance.) You will learn exercises that you can do at home, in the gym, and on the go to reshape your body, prevent injury, and become fit.

In Chapter 10, you will discover nine new circuits, called the 20 Minutes to Burn exercise bricks, each of which is designed to work out one body area. And then you will learn how to deliberately combine these bricks into a 20-, 40-, or 60-minute daily workout, and strategically embark on a Six-Week Jump Start to Mobility Plan.

As we cover these key, actionable topics, we will also examine in the remainder of the book the common barriers to your ability to stay moving, such as wear and tear and injuries that might sidetrack you. We will discuss nutrition basics, how to set realistic goals, and strategies for establishing the critical mental edge you need for success. We wrap up with sources of information about good equipment and organizations that offer access to specialized health professionals and resources.

Continue with me. Take the time to invest in your physical future by reading along with me and making a plan. You, too, can be inspiring—to yourself, to your family, to your friends, and even to those strangers who will wonder how you mastered fitness after 40.

HOME**WORK**

You have to recognize where you're starting from to be able to move toward your goal. Find a sheet of paper and take a few minutes to get to know yourself with this brief interview:

- Who (or what) do you believe controls your potential for health and aging? Is it you? Your choices? Your genetics? Your environment?
- What factors have been keeping you from living the fit life you desire? Write down some of these barriers.
- Are there any things that prevent you from taking the steps toward fitness after 40? If so, write down the excuses that you find yourself making over and over again.

Look over your list. Are these barriers and excuses things you cannot control, or can you do something now to clear some of them out of your way? Identify one or two of the issues you raised above that you can change this week. Can you rearrange your schedule? Walk to work or to the store instead of drive? Take the clothes off your exercise equipment at home? Do them!

"Through a combination of scientific training, disciplined diet, and advanced sports medicine, they [mature athletes] are overturning immutable laws of biology. . . . The new old pros are busy making 40 the new 30."

—John Hanc, author of
The Coolest Race on Earth

CHAPTER **TWO**

2

The New Science of Aging

I love telling inspirational stories about my patients and masters athletes who have decided to F.A.C.E. their futures and live the lives they imagined. I also love studying these masters athletes because they are enthusiastic and insightful research participants. In addition, I do not believe that our current literature on aging captures what our bodies are capable of if we commit to aging actively. This chapter summarizes some of the exciting research my colleagues and I have performed to investigate what our bodies are capable of if we eliminate the variable of inactivity. You may be surprised and delighted by what you read!

Aging does *not* inherently involve an inevitable decline from vitality to frailty. This commonly held belief is actually a myth. You are *not* destined for frailty as you age. You can be vital, active, joyful, and mobile long into the foreseeable future.

Why, then, do people believe this myth? I contend that you are not playing as hard as you once did because you are not playing as hard as you once did. Did you get that? To stay strong and vital, you must play hard and challenge your body like you did when you were young in years. Your body is a dynamic and masterful adapter capable of consistent mobility throughout your life span if you can stave off many of the changes and "slowing down" that you might have just assumed were inevitable aspects of aging.

Today, it is not unusual for professional athletes in their forties to play prominent roles in their teams' successes. From professional baseball and ice hockey players, to triathletes, Ultimate Fighters, and the crowds of amateur masters athletes who fill our streets, fields, and arenas (just to name a few), we are witnessing an amazing aging of the best of the best.

How is this possible? Isn't the human body genetically programmed to slow down? One of my all-time favorite sportswriters, John Hanc, in an article for *Best Life* magazine (in which he interviewed me), puts it very well:

> It's as though 21st-century professional athletes and weekend warriors are living out the Benjamin Button fantasy: Through a combination of scientific training, disciplined diet, and advanced sports medicine, they are overturning immutable laws of biology, and they are reversing, or at least fighting to a draw, the aging process. The new old pros are busy making 40 the new 30.

> The truth behind the headlines, while encouraging, is complicated. Overall, athletic performance clearly declines with age. At the same time, late-career athletic productivity is showing an unprecedented rise.

As a clinician and scientist, I wanted to really look at what our bodies are capable of. I set out to prove that with a lifetime of mobility, we can actually preserve our bodies and stave off the degrading effects of sedentary living, including some of the more than 33 chronic diseases included in Sedentary Death Syndrome, which literally suck the life out of vital people.

I began studying masters athletes because these regular people (who, like you and me, are not paid professional athletes) invest every day in their mobility. Studying them removes the variable of sedentary living and lets us see exactly what our bodies are capable of if we remain mobile and fit after 40.

My aim as an orthopaedic surgeon is to teach you about yourself and to demystify the mysterious changes occurring within. In fact, I believe that the more information I can give you and the better you understand yourself, the better you will make key decisions. This is true for my patients and for you. What you are about to read summarizes the series of studies I have performed on masters athletes and is some of the very same information I give my patients every day.

DOES LIVING LONG MEAN SLOWING DOWN?

In a sense, your cells are immortal and ageless. They have the capacity to divide and renew themselves. As you age, however, this regeneration capacity slows; your tissues become stiffer and perform less efficiently. There are many examples in nature, from insects to humans, of decreased performance with increased age. Because of this overall slowdown, your physical prowess changes over time. But what part of slowing down is the result of inactivity, and what part results purely from the biology of aging? Is there a constant biologic rate of decline in your physical abilities independent of any additional health factors?

To answer the question of how fast we age, we need to look at people who are models of healthy musculoskeletal aging, such as Senior Olympians. These athletes maintain a high level of functional capacity and quality of life throughout their life spans and may represent the truest measure of pure biologic aging without the variable of disuse.

So I pose the question again: What part of slowing down is accredited to the inescapable effects of biology? To find an answer, I analyzed track athletes, ages 50 to 85, who were participating in the 2001 National Summer Senior Games.[1] As expected, with age, running times slowed somewhat in all distances from the 100-meter dash to the 10,000-meter run. Performance decline was slow and linear until people reached the age of 75, when the time it took for them to run their given distance (100 meters to 10,000 meters) increased sharply, indicating that performance was dropping precipitously. When I discussed these findings with the Senior Olympians, they said they recognized the change. Many thought, however, that their own performance had just changed with time—not the performance of all athletes their age.

Each year from age 50 to 75, performance times slowly crept up by less than 2 percent per year. When race times are plugged into statistical tests, the differences between runners at different ages were not significant until we reach the 75-year-old age group. At this point, the rate of decline per year increased to almost 8 percent per year. (See Figure 1.)

Figure 1. Change in performance with age for Senior Olympians.

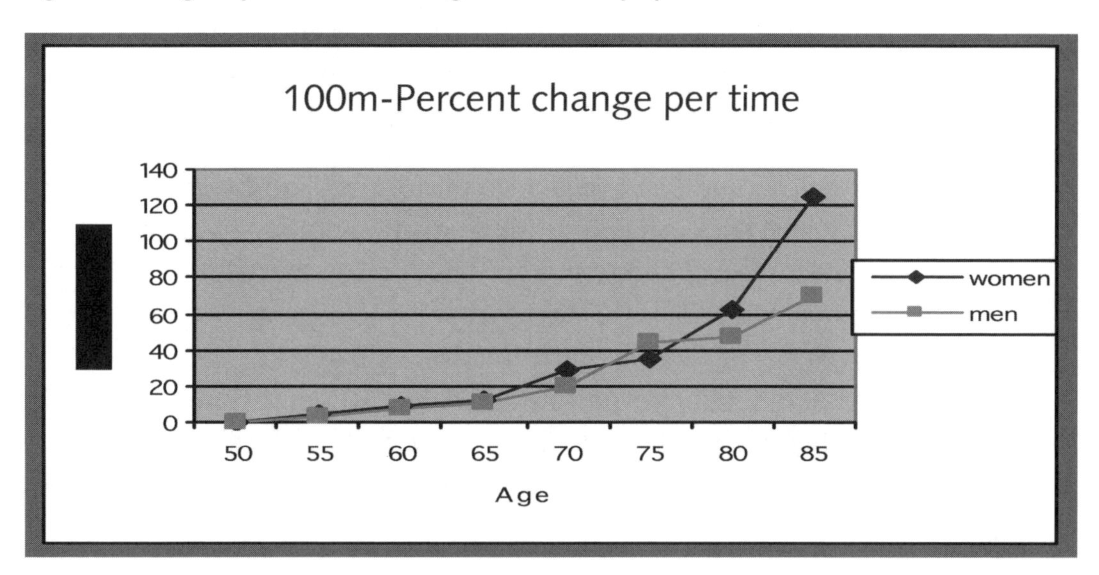

Source: Vonda J. Wright, M.D., and Brett C. Perricelli, M.D., "Age-Related Rates of Decline in Performance Among Elite Senior Athletes," *American Journal of Sports Medicine* 36(3), 2008.

In track athletes, then, performance times are well maintained until age 50 and then they modestly decline until 75, at which point performance becomes markedly slower. This finding suggests that if disuse and disease are eliminated as contributing variables, you should be able to maintain a high level of functional independence until at least 75. Loss of functional independence before age 75, therefore, is most likely the result of disease, disuse, genetic predisposition, or destructive lifestyle habits.

Sustained performance is also seen in swimming, triathlon, cycling, and weight lifting. Hirofumi Tanaka and Douglas R. Seals, two of the leaders in exercise physiology research, have published many studies on peak exercise performance in swimming across the life span.[2] They compare peak performance between long-distance (1500-meter) and short-distance (50-meter) races and have found only modest declines in peak performance between the ages of 40 and 70. After 70, swimming performance declines were exponential, as I found with runners.

Tanaka and Seals have also performed side-by-side comparisons of swimming and running, examining how peak performances corresponded with age. They found that although both groups maintained their performance with only modest curvilinear declines in performance until age 70, the runners' overall reduction of performance was 30 percent more with advancing age. This means that our performance is not only based on our own physiology and work ethic but also on the task we undertake.

Triathlon is an exploding sport. According to the Sports and Fitness Industry Association, there are nearly 3 million triathletes in the United States, with 43 percent in the age divisions that include people 40 and above. Romuald Lepers, Beat Knechtle, and Paul Stapley found improvements in performance times in both men and women in the 19 years between the ages of 40 and 59.[3] Female masters-age triathletes and male triathletes over 44 improved their swimming, cycling, running, and overall performance times during the last 25 years. Overall, peak triathlon performance declined 13 percent per decade for men and 15 percent per decade for women until the age of 70. Cycling performance declined less than that for swimming and running.

Sustained peak performance with active aging is also witnessed in weight lifters. David Meltzer measured a 1.0–1.5 percent deterioration rate of lifting capacity each year, with accelerated decline after the age of 70.[4] The absolute differences between the weight lifters and controls were such that an 85-year-old weight lifter was as powerful as a 65-year-old control subject. This would, therefore, represent an apparent age advantage of approximately 20 years for the weight lifters.

These three studies of peak performance across life spans of active aging indicate that amateur athletes are able to maintain much of their youthful athletic performance by investing every day in their mobility and performance. They were able to "play hard" because they continued to "play hard."

THE IMPORTANCE OF "BASHING YOUR BONES"

After asking the question "How fast do we age?" I was interested as a bone doctor in whether chronic mobility could keep our bones strong. In two studies, I found that the masters athletes in the Senior Olympics did maintain their bone density at a high percentage into their seventh and eighth decades. Moreover, I found, high-impact sports—or as I like to call it, "bashing your bones"—was as important as age, sex, family history, and weight in determining bone health. These studies proved that frailty is not inevitable and chronic mobility can go a long way toward preserving bone health.

I can tell you that bone health is not something many of us think about regularly until we break one—and then, it is all we think about. You want your bones to live as long as you do, but bone weakness (osteoporosis and osteopenia) is silent and hidden until we fall and break a bone, and then it can be deadly. Previous fracture is the Number 1 predictor of future fracture. Osteoporosis is often thought of as a condition mainly affecting women. However, 2 million men in the United States have osteoporosis. The results can mean fragility, decrease in height, lack of independence, and even loss of life.

When a person falls and breaks a hip, there is a 6.3 percent chance that he or she will die in the hospital. Of the 93.7 percent who make it home, one-third die in the first year after the fall. (The risks increase if the person is older, male, and living in a long-term care facility.) Of the two-thirds who survive, 50 percent never return to their pre-fracture function and require help with daily activities. This means they may not be able to live in the home where they raised their families or return to the life they love.

These statistics are sobering, but our studies prove that your daily investment in impact exercise can go a long way toward keeping you fracture-proof.

I FOUND THE FOUNTAIN OF YOUTH

Today it seems as if many of us are following Juan Ponce de León's life passion, traveling many miles and searching for that one elixir (pill, diet, cream, and so forth) that will revitalize our youth. Frankly, it is much more likely that the traveling itself kept Señor Ponce de León young—and not any kind of "magic water."

A large long-term cross-sectional observation study recently reported that even minimal amounts of mobility decreases our overall mortality rate and risk of cardiovascular disease. Researchers from New Orleans reported in the *Journal of the American College of Cardiology* that as little as 30 to 60 minutes of jogging a week lowers the risk of early death from all causes by 30 percent and from death by heart attack or stroke by 45 percent.[5]

So you don't have to be a marathon runner to make a significant life-preserving impact on your health. No! On a genetic level, you are programmed to move. Your body does not know whether you are hunting and gathering right outside your cave or traveling long distances to find food. Your body simply knows it is moving. And moving keeps the genes that transcribe for health, mobility, muscle, and bone health turned on. If your body perceives that you are just sitting around, it thinks you are waiting for winter to be over and your metabolism goes into hibernation mode.

How does mobility itself help you retain your youthful vigor? One important way is by maintaining your lean muscle mass.

One of the biggest complaints people report about the aging process is feeling weak. They can't carry as much, as far; they get tired earlier. One reason this may occur is due to the loss of lean muscle mass. Many population-based studies have shown that lean muscle loses cells and muscle fibers with age and becomes stiff. This loss of lean muscle mass, or sarcopenia, results in the loss of power and endurance. In sedentary populations, Walter Frontera and his colleagues reported declines in muscle area of up to 15 percent per decade between ages 50 and 75, resulting in three to four times more disability.[6] In addition, the Health ABC Study of a cohort of people ages 70 to 79 found that sedentary lean muscle becomes grossly infiltrated with fat.[7] In other words, abnormal amounts of fat build up between muscle fibers and even within the cells themselves—like the marbling of a beefsteak.

What happens to your muscle when you are chronically (regularly) active and moving? My colleagues and I decided to answer that question by studying amateur masters athletes who exercised four to five times per week.[8] By taking cross-sectional pictures of the athletes' upper legs with an MRI scanner, I was able to track the amount of lean muscle mass and the amount of fat infiltration in active muscle. What I found was astounding.

Chronic mobility preserves lean muscle mass, prevents fatty infiltration of the muscle, and keeps muscles strong. There *is* a fountain of youth—and the elixir is mobility! The best way to grasp the profound effect of mobility on lean muscle mass is to see it.

The first image in Figure 2 is a cross-sectional MRI of the thigh of a 40-year-old triathlete. It is like a lean flank steak. It has gorgeous muscle structure, no fat infiltration of the muscle, and minimal subcutaneous (under the skin) fat. The second picture is a cross-sectional MRI of the thigh of a sedentary 74-year-old man. Profoundly different, right? It shows poor muscle structure, highly marbled fat infiltration, and a thick layer of subcutaneous fat. It looks more like a rump roast than a flank steak. Now look at the third image. This is the punch line. This MRI shows the thigh of a chronically active 70-year-old man, a triathlete. His thigh is like a lean flank steak—gorgeous muscle structure, low fat infiltration, and minimal subcutaneous fat. The bonus is that the chronically active man's quadriceps muscles remain strong. In my study, there was no statistical difference in strength in any age group until age 60 and then no additional difference until the last age group at 80.

SEDENTARY LIVING ITSELF SLOWS US DOWN

Unfortunately, I see the ravages of a sedentary lifestyle in my patients. I have had many chronologically younger patients (in their fifties and early sixties) who appear and feel old before their years. Research has shown that sedentary people decline twice as fast as their active counterparts.

Jim is a 51-year-old accountant. At 5'9", he has a large belly (a big risk factor for heart disease and diabetes) and admitted

Figure 2. Chronic exercise preserves lean muscle mass in masters athletes.

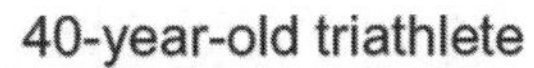

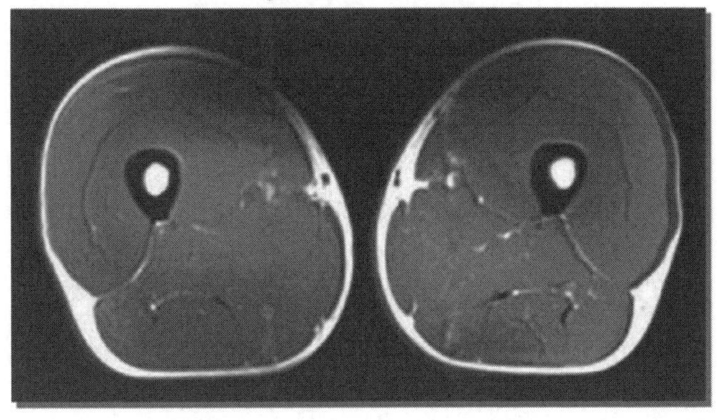

74-year-old sedentary man

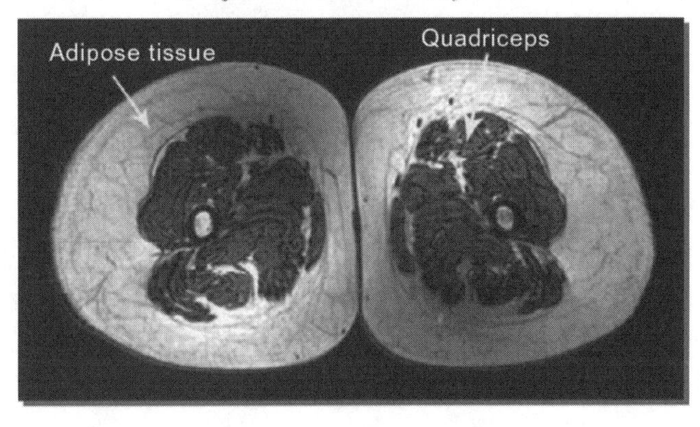

70-year-old triathlete

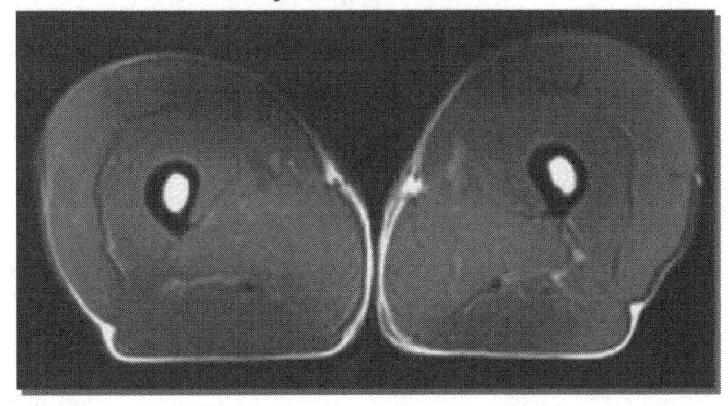

Source: Andrew P. Wroblewski, Francesca Amati, Mark A. Smiley, Bret Goodpaster, and Vonda Wright, "Chronic Exercise Preserves Lean Muscle Mass in Masters Athletes," *Physician and Sports Medicine* 39(3) (2011).

that although he had been an athlete in college, the only exercise he gets now is walking to the men's room and the company cafeteria. He came to see me because he had neck and back pain, which he attributed entirely to his occupation. In addition to musculoskeletal problems, inactive patients like Jim typically also have high blood pressure, obesity, and type II diabetes; they become short of breath after simple activities. I treat their immediate orthopaedic problems, but I also encourage them to take the time to make a daily investment in their health by becoming physically active. I emphasize that when they are older and perhaps disabled, they will surely look back at the missed opportunity they have now for prevention.

One of the most satisfying aspects of my practice is when I convince Jim (and the many others like him) to get off the couch and invest daily in his physical health by becoming active. At times, there are barriers to people becoming active, but often people just need some encouragement, education, handholding, or even a swift kick in the right direction to start down a path that will benefit them greatly. I began a program for my patients that does all four of these things. PRIMA Start is for adult-onset exercisers or people getting back into the game after a long break. It takes people from the couch to a 5K walk/run in just 12 weeks. Through twice-weekly meetings and group exercise sessions, many of my patients have lowered their body fat, increased their fitness level, learned the components of well-rounded fitness after 40, and set and achieved fitness goals for the first time in years!

It is interesting to observe the difference physical activity can make in the lives of my patients. It always makes my day to see patients like Rita, a tall, slim, 45-year-old caterer who whisked into my office one day. She regaled me with tales of her last run, bike, and swim with great enthusiasm. She came to PRIMA Start with the goal of getting rid of her knee pain so she could compete in an upcoming marathon. Often I glance over the medical histories of patients like Rita only to find that, even in their sixties and seventies, they are taking no medication. If they have ever been hospitalized, it was years ago when they had their children. This is very different from the histories of my patients who have lived sedentary lives. Such people usually have started suffering from health problems in their late forties or early fifties, including high blood pressure, high cholesterol, and (depending on their weight) the onset of diabetes. All of these health problems can be modified with daily exercise, which is why I spend so much time talking to my patients about fitness. It is really the best way to control some aspects of your future health.

AGE-RELATED FACTORS

Your first step in becoming physically fit is understanding the multiple age-related factors—such as heart, lung, and muscle strength—that can contribute to your ability to care for yourself and your family as well as participate in athletics.

The factors include:

- Your ability to train intensely, your reaction time, and your joint mobility
- Your skeletal size
- Your body fat composition
- Your anaerobic and aerobic power supply
- Your ability to recover
- Your strength, endurance, and coordination

According to Wojtek Jan Chodzko-Zaiko, a professor of kinesiology at the University of Illinois, "Of all the variables limiting performance in the older athlete, physiological changes aren't enough by themselves to prevent him from staying near the top of his game. It's not as if some light goes out in the body at 43, or at any other age. Athletes who remain competitive past the age of 40 do so because of a complex set of reasons, not because of the number of fast-twitch fibers." (These fibers, discussed later in the chapter, are responsible for muscle power.)

Let's consider some of these factors.

FACTORS CONTRIBUTING TO A DECLINE IN PEAK PERFORMANCE WITH AGING

Many factors contribute to declines in peak performance. Some can be modified with chronic intense mobility.

- Heart rate decreases 10bpm (beats per minute) each decade.
- Lean muscle mass declines.
- IMAT (intramuscular adipose tissue, or fat in the muscles) increases in sedentary people.
- Fast-twitch muscle declines.
- Lung function decreases.
- Anabolic hormones such as testosterone decline.
- Quality of neuronal pathways (the nerve pathways between your brain and muscles) becomes less efficient.
- Lactate threshold (the point of exercise intensity where the body starts accumulating the substance lactate in the blood) declines.
- Exercise economy (the motion and ease of movement of muscles) declines.

- VO2 max (the maximum volume of oxygen available for energy production, which is discussed in greater detail shortly) performance declines up to 10 percent per year in sedentary people.
- Cardiac output (how much blood comes out of your heart with each contraction), absolute heart rate, and oxygen uptake all decline.
- Time for training diminishes, as a result of life commitments.

ENDURANCE CAPACITY: IT'S ALL ABOUT MOVING OXYGEN

As you are reading this, hold your breath. It will be easy at first, but as you flip the pages, you will begin to feel the involuntary hunger for air, which is triggered by your brain stem. This hunger will grow and grow until your body demands that you take a gasp of air. Your brain is serious about making sure that you get enough oxygen, and if you don't take a breath, you will pass out, which is your body's way of overriding your voluntary withholding of oxygen.

Oxygen is just that important to every cell in your body. Without it, your cells can't make energy, and their metabolism is less effective. You switch from being a highly efficient energy-making machine to being 16 times less efficient and generating a lot of lactic acid (which is what builds up in your muscles and makes you sore). Without sufficient oxygen, you perform less effectively.

Getting oxygen from the outside air to inside your cells takes collaboration among your lungs, heart, arteries, and the muscle cells they feed. As you age, the efficiency of oxygen delivery, and therefore your ability to perform at a peak level, shifts. The changes in performance with aging are attributed to lower lactate threshold, lower exercise economy/efficiency, and lower VO2 max. VO2 max is the most important of these factors.

As stated above, VO2 max is the maximum volume (V) of oxygen (O2) available for energy production via the oxidative pathway (the highly efficient system of metabolism in which energy is produced). VO2 max is dependent upon your heart rate, cardiac output, and tissue oxygen uptake (how much oxygen is taken into the tissues).

Reductions in VO2 max are believed to be the primary reason for a decline in functional endurance with aging. Interestingly, scientists believe that part of the decline in VO2 max is due to lower energy, intensity, and time spent in activity or training.

How does aging change the efficiency of your heart and lungs in delivering oxygen? Let's find out.

Your Heart: The Pump That Moves the Oxygen

What an amazing piece of engineering your heart is! Essentially, it comprises complex pumps that are able to adapt your blood pressure, blood flow, and blood volume to provide your body with all the blood it needs. Over 50 years, an average of 80 beats per minute (which is the average heart rate) equals 2.1 billion heartbeats. It is little wonder that your heart changes with age. As you grow older, your heart adjusts. These adjustments come with trade-offs, leaving your heart more vulnerable to disease and other problems. Your maximum heart rate, heart muscle contractility (the ability of cardiac muscle fibers to contract), and the amount of blood coming out of your heart into your body (called stroke volume) all decline with age.

In general, without a preventive program, your heart will simply not function as well once you get older. Here are some statistics:

- In people ages 65 to 74, 40 percent of deaths are from heart disease. For those over age 80, the figure is 60 percent.
- Typically, in your twenties, your maximum heart rate (MaxHR) with exertion is between 180 and 200 beats per minute. At age 80, it is down to 145bpm.
- A 20-year-old's heart typically outputs (pumps out) 3.5 to four times as much blood as its resting capacity. An 80-year-old can output only twice the resting capacity.

You can counteract or slow many of the changes the heart experiences by exercise, blood pressure control, emotional stress reduction, and diet. Improving your heart function is one of the main objectives of continuing to exercise or beginning to exercise after 40.

When your blood pressure increases, your heart adjusts by pumping harder. This is because your arteries—the blood vessels that take oxygen-rich blood away from your heart and deliver it to the rest of your body—become stiffer and less flexible with age. This stiffening and loss of flexibility causes blood pressure to increase. Researchers have noted that the wall of the left ventricle of the heart becomes thicker with age. This thickening allows your heart to pump more strongly against the resistance of stiff arteries.

All these adjustments, however, leave your heart more vulnerable. Your arteries become less able to respond to changes in the amount of blood pumped through them. Thus, blood pressure may be higher in older people than in younger people.

As your heart ages, it also becomes less able to respond rapidly to chemical messages from your brain. The result is that the body cannot exercise as long or as intensely as when you were younger. This shows up as shortness of breath with less work—a sign that oxygen-rich blood is not moving fast enough through your body because your lungs are trying to breathe in more oxygen.

The heart of a healthy 70-year-old has 30 percent fewer cells than the heart of a 20-year-old. When heart cells die, the other cells must stretch and grow to stay connected. An older person's heart cells may thus be up to 40 percent larger than a younger person's.

It sounds all bad, but it is not. Exercise can keep your heart younger and more efficient. My 75-year-old dad's resting heartbeat is in the mid-50s, compared with the average resting heart rate of 80. The more fit you are, the lower your average resting heart rate will be because your heart is more efficient and pumps more blood volume with each beat. This means that even at my dad's age, the exercise he has done keeps his heart in shape.

How Fit Is Your Heart Now?

One way to measure how fit your heart is right now is to look at the maximum amount of oxygen (VO2 max) your body is capable of taking up and using in your muscles. Oxygen use declines 5–15 percent per decade after age 25. The greatest portion of this decline is the result of changes in cardiac output (the amount of blood that is pumped from your heart in one minute). As training levels or activity in general declines, so does the VO2 max. (Men and women have relatively similar rates of VO2 max decline.) This does not mean that the hearts of masters athletes do not adapt to high-intensity exercise: Hawaiian Ironmen, for example, between the ages of 58 and 71 show the same heart changes (lower resting heart rates, larger left ventricles, and higher blood return volumes) as their younger counterparts. (Note that the age-predicted heart rate maximum decreases one beat per year after the age of 10. Each year we age, our hearts are capable of beating less quickly. This is due to a slower time of contraction and a longer rest period between beats.)

The good news is that physical training can maintain cardiac output and improve your body's ability to provide and use oxygen. How much it improves depends a lot on how you exercise. Intense endurance exercise, performed throughout one's life, has been found to cut the decline in VO2 max in half. When physical exercise is begun later in life, it can lower the loss of maximum heart rate, but it cannot increase heart rate by lowering contraction time.

The take-home message of all this: Keeping your heart fit through regular aerobic exercise helps maintain the amount of blood your heart is able to pump out with each heartbeat and deliver to your body.

Your Arteries: A Highway for Oxygen

To understand why aging is so closely linked to cardiovascular disease—and ultimately to find the causes and develop cures for this group of diseases—it is essential to understand what is happening to your arteries during normal aging (that is, aging in the absence of disease). This understanding has moved forward dramatically in the past decades, according to Richard J. Hodes, the director of the National Institute on Aging. He points out:

> While we know a great deal about cardiovascular disease and its risk factors, new areas of research are beginning to shed further light on the link between aging and the development and course of the disease. For instance, scientists at

> the National Institute on Aging . . . are paying special attention to certain age-related changes that occur in the arteries and their influence on cardiac function. Many of these changes, once considered a normal part of aging, may put people at increased risk for cardiovascular disease.

Arteries are the tubes that carry blood away from your heart to your lungs and to all the other tissues of the body. Arteries are made of muscle, and like other muscles in our bodies, they tend to stiffen with age. Stiffening or hardening of the arteries also accompanies a high-fat diet and smoking. In addition, as our blood vessels age, they become narrower. This causes the blood pressure to increase because the heart must work harder to pump the same amount of blood through a smaller space. The heart compensates for this by becoming bigger.

The hardening of the arteries makes the heart's job of pumping blood through them more difficult, since hard arteries are narrower and more resistant to flow. Soft, supple arteries do not show up on X-rays, but hard, calcified arteries look like shadowy bone. It is not uncommon for me to take an X-ray of a person's knee and see outlines of the arteries coursing down her legs. Hardening of the arteries is not inevitable: Many studies show that exercise can make arteries more pliable. Supple arteries are not only good for heart health; they also keep blood flowing to the brain and are good for sexual performance.

Your Lungs: The Gateway That Delivers the Oxygen into Your Blood

Every athlete gets out of breath when he runs fast. How soon you start panting is a measure of your fitness.

I remember a patient named Donna. Overweight and out of shape, she had difficulty completing the flexibility exercises we were teaching her because she would get short of breath. As the weeks went by, however, her body adapted to the new demands she was placing on it, and she began walking around the track with less distress. Each week, she added a little more distance and gradually could finish a mile, then two, then three comfortably.

Getting the oxygenated blood into your heart is one component of feeding your tissue, but first you actually have to breathe air to get oxygen into your blood. This is the role of your lungs. Moving air from the outside world to inside you is a simple matter of rolling downhill. What I mean by this is that oxygen will diffuse, or go where it is needed most, when it enters the small air sacs in your lungs. Thus, when air is breathed in, the oxygen "sees" blood in the body that needs it. The oxygen attaches itself to the red blood cells to be carried to the waiting tissue. Anything that makes the lungs more stiff (such as age, smoking, or asthma) therefore prevents oxygen from entering the lungs, which in turn decreases delivery to the blood.

It takes more energy to breathe as you get older. This is because the amount of air your lungs can hold decreases by about 250 milliliters (8.5 ounces, about the size of a teacup) per decade. From age 20 to 70, your maximum breathing capacity (called vital capacity) typically declines by about 40 percent.

In addition, the elasticity (the give of the lung tissue) decreases. There is also a decline in the number of lung capillaries (small blood vessels) and the quality of perfusion (oxygen exchange). Essentially, your lungs get stiffer and hold air and exchange oxygen for carbon dioxide less efficiently. The Number 1 thing you can do for your lungs as you age is stop smoking.

Your Muscles: The Strength of the Machine

It's all good to have efficient fuel (oxygen) delivery, but what your body can do with it, once the oxygen is delivered, depends on the integrity of your muscles. Age-related changes to muscles and tendons have a great impact on your activities of daily living as well as your ability to participate in sports. They affect a muscle's power (the ability to move quickly) and its overall strength.

The changes seen in our muscles as we age are largely the result of loss of muscle cells, decreased size of muscle fibers, and increased muscle stiffness. Most of the muscle changes seen with aging are caused by the loss of lean muscle mass (sarcopenia). We lose lean muscle mass beginning around age 50. By age 80, we have lost 50 percent of our lean muscle mass. People who are sedentary lose 15 percent of their muscle mass each decade between ages 50 and 70, and 30 percent per decade after age 70.

Our age-related muscle atrophy results from the shrinking of what are called type II (fast-twitch) muscle fibers. These fibers, which are responsible for muscle power, actually may shrink by 30 percent. This may be one reason that aged sprinters have markedly shorter stride lengths (40 percent shorter) and require a significantly higher number of strides to cover the same distance as younger sprinters. Not only do we lose lean muscle mass but studies of sedentary 70- to 79-year-olds have found that the muscles actually become replaced with fat. This is all true unless we do something about it.

Muscles become harder to move and more stiff with age. Loss of water and maturation of the structural components of your tendons and ligaments cause them to become stiff. This is due to changes in the muscle composition as well as the way the individual muscle fibers cross-link during contraction. Stiff muscles are more susceptible to muscle injury.

If you need more motivation to keep your muscles moving, Swedish and Finnish researchers biopsied a muscle that extends the knee (called the vastus lateralis) in 18- to 84-year-old male sprinters. They found that the sprint-trained athletes did experience the typical aging-related reduction in the size of fast-twitch fibers, which play a role in the decline in explosive force required for sprinting. The muscle characteristics, however, were preserved at a high level in the oldest runners, underlining the favorable impact of sprint exercise on aging muscle.

The good news is that old muscle has the capacity to grow in size (called hypertrophy), just as young muscle does. In a classic study of frail elderly people, Maria Fiatarone, formerly of Tufts University, found that weight training (consisting of eight repetitions at 80 percent of the maximum weight a person could lift once, three times per week) resulted in a 5 percent increase in strength per training day.[9] Other researchers found that untrained elders can increase their rate of muscle building after two weeks of moderate weight training. If even frail 90-year-old men can increase their strength, then you can, too.

Disuse atrophy may be another reason we lose both type I (slow-twitch endurance fibers) and type II (fast-twitch power muscle fibers) over the years. High-intensity training in masters athletes leads to muscle hypertrophy (or growth) and increased size of both type I and type II muscle fibers.

A study of masters athletes who engage in exercise for fitness (running and swimming without weight training) found that they had muscle composition similar to age-matched sedentary people, whereas those athletes who also participated in strength straining (such as weight training) had muscle fiber composition similar to control subjects who were 40 years their junior. Other studies show that differences in muscle composition between masters and youth runners is also because of differences in training programs, with similar regimens resulting in similar muscle composition.

The point of all these studies is that exercise not only feels good and makes your muscles look more fit but that staying active helps your muscles actually regain or maintain their more youthful makeup.

In addition to caring for masters athletes, I also have a laboratory where we investigate muscle and tendon aging with the goals of finding ways to make aging tissues heal faster. My research partner, Fabrisia Ambrosio, and I were recently discussing some experiments she had performed. It appears that aging muscle cells can be made to behave more youthfully by using simple rehabilitation methods such as electrical stimulation. Dr. Ambrosio found that when muscle stem cells are harvested from old mice that had previously been exercised using electrical stimulation (a very common current rehabilitation method that stimulates both power and endurance muscle fibers), these old cells began to act more like muscle stem cells from young mice. It is exciting to think that exercise could actually change the very behavior of old cells! Another collaborator, Yong Li, found that muscle stem cells harvested from the muscles between the ribs of old mice also acted like young cells. This makes sense if exercise keeps muscle cells acting young because there is never a time when the muscles between your ribs are not exercising and moving to keep you breathing. In our laboratory, it appears that exercise could be the Fountain of Youth—all the way down to the cellular level!

A few years ago, I was about to see a patient with a colleague who specializes in trauma. I read something on the chart about a 70-year-old male who had been involved in a motorcycle crash having shoulder pain. I paused as I walked into the room and met Hank, a man with muscles almost like Arnold

Schwarzenegger's. In his retirement from his first career as a business executive, Hank had decided to make his second career staying at peak performance and health. Now I am not suggesting that we all have to look like Arnold to be fit, but I am suggesting that an intentional approach to health, and in this case musculoskeletal fitness, can maintain our physical function regardless of our date of birth.

EXERCISE ECONOMY: HOW IT ALL FITS TOGETHER

So far, we've seen that oxygen is being delivered and that muscles use the oxygen to provide power and endurance for motion. How much motion and the ease of movement produced are termed *exercise economy*.

Decreased joint motion, coordination, and flexibility contribute significantly to declines in exercise economy. As discussed, aged sprinters have markedly shorter stride lengths than their younger counterparts and may take up to twice the number of strides to cover the same distance. While part of this may be the effect of lost muscle strength and power, the other important component is joint flexibility. Connective tissue, such as ligaments and tendons, are inherently stiffer with aging. This is the result of an age-related loss of tissue water content and maturation of the collagen in ligaments and tendons. In addition, many systemic diseases (i.e., those affecting the whole body) can make these tissues stiffer. As a result, joint motion decreases. For instance, knee motion decreases with aging. It is 120 to 130 degrees when we are in our forties and drops to 95 degrees when we are in our seventies and eighties.

Maintaining supple tissues by paying attention to stretching and flexibility is very important. Simply put, flexible soft tissue performs better than stiff tissue! Flexibility also maintains the stretch/reflex response of muscle and, thereby, boosts speed. Finally, stretching may reduce delayed exercise soreness.

In addition to the areas we have already discussed, there are several other important physiologic changes that occur with aging. They involve cartilage, bones, tendons, body fat, and the neuromuscular system.

Your Cartilage: Slicker than Ice, but Fragile

Aging cartilage is a big problem in the general population, but it can be especially vexing for the masters athlete who has no time or inclination to be slowed down by the pain or swelling that often accompanies cartilage that is "running out." Keeping cartilage healthy is a real balancing act for mature athletes. Inactivity and disuse atrophy can decrease the health of cartilage, causing softening, fissuring, and potential mechanical compromise. On the other hand, high-energy, high-impact activity on degenerated cartilage can cause increased wear. If you are a jogger or basketball player over 40, you must take this into consideration by listening to your body and the pain messages it sends. Such messages tell you that you are tired, that there is a problem or damage, or that the soft tissue of your joint is inflamed. When you feel these signals, be smart and *stop or moderate* what you are doing. You make no gains by ignoring the pain and continuing to abuse your cartilage.

Your Bones: A Dynamic Framework

Bone is an amazing, dynamic organ that is constantly changing and remodeling itself over our life spans. It is the only organ that can heal without leaving a scar and change its shape based on the stresses it experiences. This works in both directions. When bones experience a lot of stress or load, they get stronger. When they are not used to doing heavy work, whether it is labor or exercise, they get weak.

Our bones are made of a dense outer cortex and a spongy inner matrix of boney arches and bridges called trabeculae. When we age, we lose a number of these trabeculae. After age 40, women lose bone twice as fast as men at a range of 1.5–2 percent per year. This rate increases to 3 percent per year after menopause. Loss of bone density can lead to frailty and disability because of fractures.

We conducted a study of bone density in senior athletes and found that many more women had normal bone density than weak bone. This held true in even the oldest female athletes, who were more than 80 years old. The prevalence of osteoporosis in female Senior Olympians was less than in the general population at any age. In addition, significantly fewer participants in weight-bearing sports had osteoporosis. This all goes to show that even in chronically exercising senior athletes, doing high-impact exercise such as running and jumping is better for your bones. (Of course, exercise of any kind is better for the bones than being inactive.)

Your Tendons: The Ties That Bind

Tendons are the tough cords of tissue that connect your muscles to your bones. In fact, every muscle in your body has a tendon that attaches to bone. Tendons, thus, can be large in size, such as those around your knee joints, or small, like the ones in your fingers.

Tendinitis is a painful condition that leaves the tendons irritated, swollen, and sore. It is a common condition, especially in over-40 athletes. Essentially, this inflammation occurs as the tendon develops repetitive microtears (very small tears). The pulling of the tendon between the muscle and bone is felt mostly at the tendon insertion site and at the junction of the muscle and tendon. Tendinitis results after excessive repetitive movement. Continued use without stretching causes the fibers to gradually become tighter. For example, if you play tennis, you may overuse the muscles of your elbow through hitting the ball repetitively. This strains your wrist flexors where they begin on the outside of the elbow. The most common parts of the body where tendinitis occurs are the elbow, wrist, biceps, shoulder (including rotator cuff attachments), leg, knee (patellar and quadricep), and Achilles.

Of course, the condition can vary with each person as it strikes the areas she uses most. Symptoms can vary from an achy pain and stiffness in the local area of the tendon to a burning that surrounds the whole joint around the inflamed tendon. Typically, the pain is worse during and after activity, and the tendon and joint area can become stiffer the following day.

One of the most serious tendon problems is Achilles tendinitis and rupture. (Men in their forties and fifties are especially prone to the latter.) The Achilles tendon connects the three large calf muscles to your heel. You never think about the Achilles until the slow ache you feel in the back of your leg explodes. Men who come into my office with this problem often literally say something like "It feels like someone shot me in the leg!"

Your Body Fat: The Storage System for Excess Energy

Body fat does not just hang around in unfortunate places looking for something to do. Fat is a toxic metabolic organ that pads your body and stores excess energy, releasing hormones and chemicals that change the very way your body functions.

If none of the cardiac, lung, or muscle changes we've talked about motivate you to get off the couch and get active, certainly looking buff and fit should. Many of my patients are happy that their hearts and muscles are stronger, but they are elated when they look in the mirror. Often, after a few weeks of exercise, my patients comment that their clothes are fitting more loosely. Even before they see a large difference when they step on the scale, their body composition changes to become more muscular and less fatty.

Body fat composition rises in both men and women with age, and thus the percentage of lean muscle mass declines. Typically, active men at age 20 have 12–16 percent body fat, which rises to 19–26 percent by age 60. In the same time period, body fat in women rises from 23–28 percent to 28–38 percent. As body fat rises, inactive muscles become infiltrated with fat, which leads to decreased muscle strength.

For more than 50 years, however, researchers have known that it is not only the amount of fat you have hanging around that matters but where it is hanging. If you carry fat mainly around your waist, you are more likely to develop health problems than if you carry fat mainly in your hips and thighs. This is true even if your weight falls within the normal range.

Why is fat so dangerous? Not only does fat serve as a place to store excess energy but it also functions as a hormone-making organ. According to Robert Ross of Queen's University in Ontario, Canada, fat produces many hormones that cause high blood sugar (the hormone resistin), cause high blood pressure (the hormone angiotensinogen), cause accumulation of plaque and inflammation in our arteries, and regulate our blood lipids (a type of fat). Fat around our middles (visceral fat) is much more productive than peripheral fat (the fat under our skin) and is therefore much more dangerous to our health.

When you carry your weight around your waistline, you are more likely to develop what is called metabolic syndrome. This is a dangerous condition where your waist measures greater than 40 inches if you are a man and greater than 35 inches if you are a woman and you have two of the following four cardiac risk factors: high triglycerides (blood fat), high blood sugar, high blood pressure, and low HDL (the good cholesterol). Metabolic syndrome increases the likelihood of developing type II diabetes by more than 500 percent, of having a heart attack by 300 percent, and of dying of a heart attack by 200 percent. Get out your tape measures and measure your waist now, and then let's get out and do some exercise.

A study by physiologist Cris Allan Slentz, assistant professor of medicine at Duke University, and colleagues published in the *Journal of Applied Physiology* is a prime example of the benefits of exercise alone.[10] Slentz's study included 175 men and women between the ages of 40 and 65 in North Carolina. All were overweight, inactive, and had mild to moderate cholesterol problems. The study subjects agreed to the following protocol for six months:

- The first group (the control group) stayed sedentary.
- The second group engaged in low amounts of moderate-intensity exercise (equal to walking 12 miles weekly).
- The third group participated in low amounts of vigorous-intensity exercise (equal to jogging 12 miles weekly).
- The final group pursued high amounts of vigorous-intensity exercise (equal to jogging 20 miles weekly).

Participants used treadmills, stationary bikes, and elliptical trainers. (Elliptical trainers are stationary exercise machines that allow for the same benefits as walking and running but reduce joint pressure and impact. They can be set on varying levels of intensity.) Subjects who exercised on the three types of machines were directly supervised or wore heart-rate monitors to check their workout intensity. They were also asked not to diet or change their diet during the study.

Before-and-after imaging scans of the belly were done to check visceral fat around the organs in the belly area. The results were as follows:

- Visceral fat rose by nearly 9 percent in the sedentary group.
- Visceral fat did not change with low amounts of exercise (at either intensity).
- Visceral fat dropped 7 percent, on average, in people who got a lot of vigorous exercise.

This study shows that exercise can decrease the most dangerous type of fat—the type that makes us look like we are a basketball on sticks. In Chapter 13, we discuss the apple and pear phenomenon of body composition. While there's little you can do to change the actual shape of the body that you inherited, you can decrease the visceral fat as well as change the appearance of your body, muscle, and skin.

Your Neuromuscular System: The Most Important Organ

The mind-body connection refers to the way your nerves and muscles work together. A decrease in coordination, balance, fine-motor skills, and visual-spatial orientation, as well as an increase in motor response time and altered proprioception (the sense of orientation of one's limbs in space), are all age-related changes in the neuromuscular system. Regular exercise seems to slow the rate of decline in many of these pathways.

As you were reading this chapter, you may have nodded as you recognized some of the changes you feel in your own body. You are no longer a mystery to yourself! But let's put all this talk of slowing down into perspective. Remember the Senior Olympians we talked about earlier in this chapter, whose times slowed by less than 2 percent per year until age 75, at which point their times grew dramatically longer? When you put those percentages into real performance times, you see that although performance slows, staying active and challenging the body with physical training can lead to remarkable functional capacity at any age. In 2011, the 50-year-old man who won the mile race at the National Summer Senior Games won it in 4:35! Let me repeat that: The 50-year-old winner ran the mile in 4:35! And the 70-year-old male winner ran the mile in 5:42. I do not know any sedentary 40-year-old men who can run a mile in 5:42—if they can last a mile at all. Masters athletes who invest in their health and mobility daily never cease to amaze me.

So now you know more about being an active athlete and exerciser after 40. You know that your body has gone through certain changes and that you have unique needs. Therefore, the important thing to remember is that many of the declines and changes seen with aging are more accurately attributed to a sedentary lifestyle or an incomplete approach to fitness and can be entirely prevented through proper training.

The take-home message here is that your body will change because of the biology of aging—but without the devastating factor of disuse, you are capable of remaining amazingly fast and functional as you age. Many of the changes popularly associated with aging are less the result of biology and more the result of the lifestyle choices people make as they grow older.

Let's make some healthy lifestyle choices together. In the next several chapters, I will help you apply this knowledge toward slowing the declines usually blamed on age. As a result, you will increase your vigor and enjoyment of life.

GET TO KNOW YOURSELF!

This chapter is packed with knowledge, but I encourage you to stop for a moment and get to know yourself. I encourage my patients to keep a card with the following current information so that they know the parts of their health profile they need to work on. It also serves to motivate them toward change:

- Weight
- Waist measurement (measuring at the top of your hip bones)
- Waist to hip ratio (this ratio should be around 0.8 or lower)
- Body composition (your body fat should be less than 25 percent)
- Cholesterol levels (including triglycerides, LDL, and HDL)
- Resting heart rate (take this when you first wake up in the morning)
- Blood pressure (this should be less than 120/80)
- Family history (know the diseases that have plagued your relatives)
- Bone density (especially for women over 50 and men over 70)

HOMEWORK

Take a few minutes to answer the following questions:

- How has your body changed in the last 20 years?
- What is better about your body?
- What is worse?
- Look at the "Get to Know Yourself" section. Do you know your numbers? If not, calculate them now.

After taking inventory of yourself, decide what you want to regain or change, and we will work together to move you to your best health.

NOTES

1. Wright, Vonda J., and Brett C. Perricelli, "Age-Related Rates of Decline in Performance Among Elite Senior Athletes," *American Journal of Sports Medicine* 36(3): 443–450 (2008).

2. Tanaka, Hirofumi, and Douglas R. Seals, "Dynamic Exercise Performance in Masters Athletes: Insight into the Effects of Primary Human Aging on Physiological Functional Capacity," *Journal of Applied Physiology* 95(5): 2152–2162 (2003).

3. Lepers, Romuald, Beat Knechtle, and Paul Stapley, "Trends in Triathlon Performance: Effects of Sex and Age," *Sports Medicine* 43(9): 851–863 (2013).

4. Meltzer, David E., "Body-Mass Dependence of Age-Related Deterioration in Human Muscular Function," *Journal of Applied Physiology* 80(4): 1149–1155 (1996).

5. Lee, Duck-chul, Russell R. Pate, Carl J. Lavie, Xuemei Sui, Timothy S. Church, and Steven N. Blair, "Leisure-Time Running Reduces All-

Cause and Cardiovascular Mortality Risk," *Journal of the American College of Cardiology* 64(5): 472–481 (2014).

6. Frontera, Walter R., Virginia A. Hughes, Karyn J. Lutz, and William J. Evans, "A Cross-Sectional Study of Muscle Strength and Mass in 45- to 78-Year-Old Men and Women," *Journal of Applied Physiology* 71: 644–650 (1991).

7. Goodpaster, Bret H., Catherine L. Carlson, Marjolein Visser, David E. Kelley, et al., "The Attenuation of Skeletal Muscle and Strength in the Elderly: The Health ABC Study," *Journal of Applied Physiology* 90(6): 2157–2165 (2001).

8. Wroblewski, Andrew P., Francesca Amati, Mark A. Smiley, Bret Goodpaster, and Vonda Wright, "Chronic Exercise Preserves Lean Muscle Mass in Masters Athletes," *Physician and Sports Medicine* 39(3): 172–178 (2011).

9. Fiatarone, Maria A., Elizabeth C. Marks, Nancy D. Ryan, Carol N. Meredith, Lewis A. Lipsitz, and William J. Evans, "High-Intensity Strength Training in Nonagenarians: Effects on Skeletal Muscle," *JAMA* 263(22): 3029–3034 (1990).

10. Slentz, Cris Allan, Lori B. Aiken, Joseph A. Houmard, et al., "Inactivity, Exercise, and Visceral Fat. STRRIDE: A Randomized, Controlled Study of Exercise Intensity and Amount," *Journal of Applied Physiology* 99(4): 1613–1618 (2005).

"Until we decide that we are worth the daily investment in our health, everything else is secondary. We are not *destined* to pass from the vibrancy and vitality of youth to the frailty of old age unless we *choose* to."

—Vonda Wright, M.D., at Women's Health Conversations, 2013

CHAPTER **THREE** 3

Fitness at 40, 50, 60, and Beyond

These are the best times of our lives. Sure, we are not 20 anymore, but frankly, thank God! It was a fun ride, but even if I had a free pass, I probably would not get on that roller coaster again. I hope you are nodding your head in agreement.

Each decade of experience your body gains has the potential to make you better if you are purposeful about your aging process—or each decade may lead to decreased physical, mental, and emotional function if you merely let time and gravity run their course. As you think ahead, know that your body is not merely a bad sequel to your 20-year-old self. Each decade is unique. Here are a few of my best tips for maximizing each decade.

YOUR FORTIES

Oh, I've loved my forties! It has been a decade of feeling stronger and smarter and more successful than ever before. When I first wrote *Fitness After 40*, I had just turned 40, was in the best shape of my life, had my first child, got my first real-paying job, and starting investing for my future like an adult.

For many people, the forties are "prime time"—both physically and mentally. You can be as physically strong as you ever were. Plus, you have earned the brain power and experience to push yourself toward success. In my opinion, 40 starts a vital decade that makes or breaks the next 30 years of your life as biology takes over.

In your twenties, your young tissue lets you get away with the carefree living of pure, mindless youth. By your forties, it's time to get all your body and brain ducks in a row and live purposefully. If you don't pay attention now to how you are living—what you are eating and how you challenge your body physically—you will find yourself pulling into your fifties living as a slower, dimmer, softer version of yourself. Gravity will start to take over, literally and figuratively, unless you do something about it now.

Here are my tips for maximizing this amazing decade:

- ***Get on the scale***. Nothing is more objective than your weight. It's not a judgment, it's a number. But more than that—it's a number you must record to know where you are starting and where you need to go.

- ***Measure your waist***. If your waistline has grown (or your pants are tight), it can be a sign of general weight mismanagement or hormone imbalance. Men's waists should be no larger than 40 inches, and women's no larger than 35 inches. Keeping your waist size in check minimizes your risk of chronic diseases due to belly fat.

- ***Get a baseline physical***. You should not meet your primary care doctor for the first time when you are sick. For best health, it is important to see your doctor when you are well. Get a baseline physical and have your blood checked. If you are a man, have your testosterone measured. If you are a woman, get your first mammogram. Know yourself.

- ***Start moving***. An object in motion stays in motion. Whether you are stepping away from the couch for the first time in years or maximizing your performance to get in the best shape of your life, your body craves mobility and will respond to a challenge.

- ***Save your heart***. The more sedentary you are, the harder your heart has to work to circulate the same volume of blood. Without exercise, your heart gets weaker and is able to pump less blood with each beat. On top of that, as you age, your blood vessels naturally get more narrow and stiff. This, in turn, increases the pressure your heart has to push against (it is like pushing a stone uphill). A weak heart and poor circulation is a setup for a heart attack down the line.

- ***Get control of your blood pressure***. Your blood pressure is determined by the strength of each heart contraction, the pressure from your blood vessels, and the amount of fluid in your body. When your blood pressure is high, your heart has to do a lot more work to push the same volume of blood into your body; it then grows larger and weaker. Work on controlling your blood pressure by managing stress (which makes the vessels even narrower), limiting salt intake (which causes fluid expansion in your body), and keeping your heart efficient by committing to intense aerobic exercise.

- ***Think about your life***. You've lived enough time to know yourself a little better and to be able to take an honest look at where you have been, where you want to go, and what barriers might keep you from your best health. It's time for honesty. Are you investing time every day in your health? If not, why? You are important enough to make this daily commitment to yourself.

- ***Finish this book***. I promise that if you pay attention to (and implement) the ideas in *Fitness After 40*, you *will* build a strong body and the best brain—for now and for the rest of your life.

YOUR FIFTIES

The Big 5–0. Bravo! If you were fit in your forties, you are in a great position for the next 20 years. However, even if you squandered your forties (by living as mindlessly as you did in your twenties), take heart: There is *never* an age or a skill level that impedes your body's ability to rise to the opportunity of better health and mobility. That said, your body will not dramatically transform to its best health without a little attention. Here's what you need to do:

- ***Get with the program***. If you're just picking up this book now, not to worry, but do make sure to take care of the items I mentioned doing in your forties. Especially important are getting on the scale, measuring your waist, and getting a baseline physical. Also important is taking a look at your parents' health. The diseases they are challenged with may be in your future unless you make purposeful choices to move the path of your life toward health.

- ***Take charge of your cardiovascular health***. Here is where I become a broken record. Get off the couch! Use the rest of this book to jump-start your mobility and maximize your performance. F.A.C.E. your future.

- ***Pay attention to your joints***. The wear and tear of life, weight, old sports injuries, and muscle weakness can make your joints pop, crack, and ache. Now is the time to lose any extra weight you might be carrying—because every extra pound you have around your belly means 7 to 10 pounds of extra pressure on all of your weight-bearing joints.

- ***Challenge your brain***. This is the decade when you really reap the benefits of your decades of acquiring knowledge and experience. Keep your assets sharp by challenging your brain with a new project, teaching younger people what you know, or learning a new skill.

- ***Check your bone density***. You should get your bone density and Vitamin D levels checked if you are petite, fair, and female; if you are shorter than you were in your forties; if either of your parents fell and broke a hip; or if you are in menopause. Weak bones are silent and hidden—until you break one and then it can be too late.

YOUR SIXTIES (AND BEYOND!)

The sixties are your trouble-shooting decade. The base you built in your forties and fifties is the foundation for how you function in your sixties—and beyond.

- ***Focus on your cardiovascular health***. If you did not pay attention to your heart before now, don't despair: There is still time to maintain and keep it beating strong. Meet with your doctor and get your heart checked out. Do the exercises throughout the book to jump-start your mobility. If you are still smoking, ask your doctor to help you and do whatever it takes to stop. If you have diabetes, make sure you are in tight control of the disease and are doing what you can to prevent inflammation and stroke.

- ***Pay attention to your brain***. Maximize your brain with smart nutrition (discussed in Chapter 13). Make a deliberate effort to keep learning new things and engaging in new skills. Maintain your friendships. Many studies show that a rich social life keeps your brain nimble and sharp as well as preserving a feeling of connectedness and well-being.

- ***Support your natural immune function***. Your ability to fight off colds and illnesses diminishes in this decade, and you may lose your immunity to common diseases (for which you were vaccinated in your youth). Nutrition plays a huge role in maintaining immune function and can be tricky as your gastrointestinal system absorbs less well with age. Now is the time to focus on getting enough daily protein, loading your diet with foods rich in antioxidants or with antioxidant supplements, and eating essential vitamins and micronutrients. Now more than ever, your waistline is not a wasteline.

HOME**WORK**

What decade is your body living in? Not sure? Go to www.sharecare.com/realage and take the RealAge Test, developed by my colleague Dr. Mike Roizen. I love encouraging my patients to take this test. It gives you a real sense of how the choices you are making are affecting the age of your body. That being said, you should follow the advice in this chapter for your chronological age—not your "RealAge."

"The more fit you are, the more resilient your brain becomes and the better it functions both cognitively and psychologically. If you get your body in shape, your mind will follow."

—John Ratey, M.D., author of
Spark: The Revolutionary New Science of Exercise and the Brain

CHAPTER FOUR 4

Move and Be Stronger, Smarter, and Happier!

You are designed to move! From the tips of your toes to the top of your head, every part of you becomes more healthy, vital, and active when you move. This includes your brain and your sense of happiness!

There is a truth in the adage "with age comes wisdom." The cumulative knowledge, experience, and earned judgment that you have gathered during your life gives you a tactical advantage in your forties, fifties, sixties, and beyond. Sure, some 20-year-olds and 30-year-olds may be able to think more quickly, but the data you have stored up from years of working and living gives your mature brain a rich capacity for life in prime time. It is no coincidence that most executives are at their peak in their middle years.

Your job now is to maximize your brain in the prime of your life. Remember: Mobility is mental exercise, too. A large body of medical literature draws connections between what we do with our bodies and how we both build a better brain and develop our sense of happiness. No longer do we believe that a failing mind and depression are inevitable parts of aging. With sedentary aging, these conditions pose a real and present danger, but with chronic mobility, you can change the day-to-day chemical environment of your brain and change the way you age.

John Ratey, in his book *Spark: The Revolutionary New Science of Exercise and the Brain*, says it well, which is why I opened the chapter with his quote (but I'm going to repeat it now): "The more fit you are, the more resilient your brain becomes and the better it functions both cognitively and psychologically. If you get your body in shape, your mind will follow."

I like to call this real interaction our "BlBlB connection"—body, brains, and bliss. In fact, I wrote all about it in my second book, *Guide to Thrive: Four Steps to Body, Brains, and Bliss*. It is exciting to me to realize that all the sweat around the track or workouts with my kids on the playground is giving me the best chance to stay smart and keep my memory strong.

CHRONIC MOBILITY MAKES YOU SMARTER

Many people cite physical weakness as one of the worst parts of aging, but for me, as for many of you, the thought of having a weakened mind is even scarier. I personally have experienced the kind of brain changes caused by sleep deprivation (both during my six-year residency and then after having my first child and getting "mommy brain"), but the real "weakening" of the brain that can come with sedentary aging is more scary.

I have seen this happen in my own family. When I was growing up, the matriarch who kept us all in step was my Great Aunt Ida. A retired schoolteacher, she was both tough and sweet, and she had a whole toolbox of amazing life skills—from raising animals to knowing how to crochet—that she learned as a farm child growing up in Kansas during the Great Depression. Great Aunt Ida would tell a never-ending stream of witty stories and jokes, all while wearing a big apron and commanding the room. She was bigger than life to me and my many cousins.

In the final years of her life, however, we all sadly watched as the hearty and smart farm woman became lost in her own home and stopped recognizing her own memories. To me, as an academic who has spent a lifetime building my mind, this is perhaps the biggest motivator of all for mobility. I want to build and keep my best brain as long as I live.

We are all fighting against a natural brain-aging process. Once we hit 40, our brain loses 5 percent of its volume per decade; this loss accelerates after 70. This means our brains actually shrink.

The great news is that exercise strengthens your brain's ability to learn at every age. Just like it stimulates the growth of capillaries around the heart, chronic intense exercise can cause the growth of capillaries around your brain, providing a route for the steady flow of oxygen, glucose, and hormones to reach and nurture your brain. The *eustress* (good stress) of mobility also sharpens your brain by causing adrenaline to stimulate and focus your thinking and arousal. In addition, when serotonin is released during exercise, it calms your brain. Both eustress and serotonin work to your advantage in learning new information.

Chronic mobility also feeds your brain over the long term by allowing the release of brain-derived neurotropic growth factor that allows for neuron production and repair. My colleagues at the University of Pittsburgh used a six-month program of intense exercise and compared the brain blood flow of active participants with that of sedentary controls. Not surprisingly, they found that exercising brains have better blood flow. Researchers at the University of Washington found that even after mild dementia has set in, a six-week program of exercise improved brain functions, such as planning, memory, and multi-tasking.

I am currently completing a study of masters athletes at PRIMA, with my colleagues Michael Tranovich and Emily Zhao, that looks at the effect of chronic exercise on executive function of the brain in active and sedentary people matched for age and education. Preliminary data appear to confirm that our decision-making ability, mental agility, working memory, and problem solving may all be maintained into our oldest decades when we are chronically active.

CHRONIC MOBILITY MAKES YOU HAPPIER

Chronic mobility is not just about building or maintaining our smarts, however. An equally impressive body of literature now documents the connection between mobility and happiness. When talking to audiences around the country, I often cite Jeremy Sibold of the University of Vermont, who documented the 12 hours of elevated mood we get from a short morning exercise burn.

A single bout of exercise is the best trip to the pharmacy your brain will ever get. A 20-minute intense workout releases powerful endorphins, which elevate your mood; adrenaline, which focuses your brain; dopamine and serotonin, which calm your brain, decrease anxiety, and give you a sense of well-being; and finally endocannabinoids, which alleviate your stress, pain, and anxiety.

Perhaps the most amazing effect of exercise on your brain is its ability to prevent and treat depression. Depression is a huge problem, one that increases with age. Whether it results from a purely chemical change or the inevitable evaluation we all do of our life, depression in our later years can lead to despair. Many researchers have found that exercise can be as effective as medication for treating depression. James Blumenthal and his colleagues at Duke University published an amazing study that found that exercise in conjunction with antidepressant medication dramatically decreased depression in test subjects, and the effect lasted for up to six months after the study was complete.[1]

All these data are encouraging motivators for using mobility as a tool to build a better brain and store up happiness as you age. Wow! Really exciting! If you are as motivated as I am, you may need to pause in your reading and go out to build some sweat equity in your brain by running around the block! What follows is an even more detailed look at the benefits of chronic mobility.

CHRONIC MOBILITY PROTECTS YOUR BRAIN

As part of the preparation that goes into conducting the research study I described previously, my colleagues, Emily Zhao and

Michael Tranovich, and I reviewed more than 22 years of cognitive research data to evaluate what scientists have to say about the protective effect of exercise on the brain and on mood. We published the review in 2014.[2] Some of the findings follow.

- ***Mobility keeps your brain big, and thereby smart***. Greater cardiovascular fitness seems to go hand-in-hand with better brain function, especially when it comes to maintaining brain structure. Parts of the brain responsible for memory, such as the hippocampus, increase in size with increased cardiovascular fitness. This results in better performance in memory tasks. The hippocampus, which is responsible for memory consolidation and spatial relationships, is preserved due to the release of BDNF (brain-derived neurotrophic factor).
- ***Exercise improves critical cognitive functions, including memory***. Loss of brain white matter results in cognitive impairment, dementia, and Alzheimer's disease, and is the biggest contributor to cognitive aging. The executive brain functions (specifically, planning, working memory, attention, problem solving, and verbal reasoning) are specifically controlled by a brain area called the cingula. In a cross-sectional study of people over the age of 60, those with the highest physical fitness had the best cingula structure integrity. Maintenance of the cingula predicts improved cognitive functions.
- ***The more complex the exercise is, the better it is for your brain***. If you are one of those people who can read, chew gum, talk to your friend, and run on the treadmill at the same time, you are really maximizing the benefits your brain receives from exercise. M. P. Boxtel and Wojtek Jan Chodzko-Zajko found that tasks requiring higher attention to detail or cognitive processing to complete were the most sensitive to exercise.

YOUR BRAIN QUESTIONS ANSWERED

Whenever I tell my patients about all of the trail-blazing studies being done about the body-brains-bliss connections, they initially react with excitement. Once the information settles, however, they tend to have very specific questions. Here are a few of the most common:

- ***How long do I need to exercise to save my brain?*** Whether I'm talking about building muscle or building a better brain, people always want to know how much and for how long they have to keep it up. The simple answer is moderate to intense physical exercise at least every other day . . . for the rest of your life. The crowd groans. Many studies document the rise in BDNF and hippocampus size after both six-month and one-year aerobic exercise programs and the resultant benefit to cognitive maintenance. However, one researcher, Kirk Erickson, specifically documented that for every year of hippocampal growth, you can reverse age-related brain loss by one to two years.[3]
- ***Can exercise improve my brain, even if it is already healthy?*** Yes! Give your brain two months of aerobic activity and it will give you improved memory and learning ability. Give it 90 minutes of walking a week for three months and it will pay you back with improved executive function, quality of life, and motor function. These data are true in young and old people alike.
- ***Can exercise improve my brain, even if I have a disease?*** Does exercise turn back time? Yes! Four- and six-month exercise-intervention studies found a reduced risk of age-related neurological disorders and improved cognitive function in patients with Alzheimer's disease.

We found a solid body of research supporting the role of chronic exercise on improving and maintaining cognitive function as well as on reducing the risk of dementia and neurodegenerative diseases by preserving brain volume and white matter connections. If your goal is to live long and prosper in both body and brain, the evidence is mounting that mobility is the key.

HOME**WORK**

Are you taking an active role in building a better brain? If you're not sure, do each of these three things—*today*!

1. Move your body! For the time being, it is fine to simply go out for a vigorous 30-minute walk. However, on the pages that follow, I'll offer specific exercises and a six-week plan to jump-start your mobility. Keep reading!
2. Learn something new. It can be anything! You might memorize the lyrics of a new song or master the origami steps to turn a dollar bill into a frog. Pick something fun—and once you have learned it, pick a new challenge.
3. Read a book in a genre that is out of the ordinary for you. I love biographies, but I just picked up Malcolm Gladwell's latest title to take my brain for a spin!

NOTES

1. Blumenthal, James A., Patrick J. Smith, and Benson M. Hoffman, "Opinion and Evidence: Is Exercise a Viable Treatment for Depression?" *ACSM's Health and Fitness Journal* 16(4): 14–21 (2012).

2. Zhao, Emily, Michael J. Tranovich, and Vonda J. Wright, "The Role of Mobility as a Protective Factor of Cognitive Functioning in Aging Adults: A Review," *Sports Health* 6(1): 63–69 (2014).

3. Erickson, Kirk I., Ruchika S. Prakash, Michelle W. Voss, Laura Chaddock, Liang Hu, Katherine S. Morris, Siobhan M. White, Thomas R. Wójcicki, Edward McAuley, and Arthur F. Kramer, "Aerobic Fitness Is Associated with Hippocampal Volume in Elderly Humans," *Hippocampus* 19(10): 1030–1039 (2009).

"Nothing can substitute for just plain hard work. I had to put in the time to get back. And it was a grind. . . . But I was completely committed to working out to prove to myself that I still could do it."

—Andre Agassi, winner of eight major tennis tournaments and Olympic gold medalist

CHAPTER **FIVE** 5

Giving Your Mobility a F.A.C.E.-Lift!

How do you stay *on* the road, court, and field and *out* of the doctor's office? Injury is the Number 1 reason active people stop moving and climb back on the couch and one of the many reasons, besides time, cited by people who don't move for their sedentary lifestyle.

In the first edition of *Fitness After 40*, I introduced my "doctor-proven" method for moving your after-40 body. It's called "F.A.C.E-ing Your Future." Most days my mind feels 26, but since I'm in my late forties, my body needs a total body and well-rounded approach to maximizing performance and minimizing injury. So does yours.

My approach to fitness after 40 is to *F.A.C.E. your future!* F.A.C.E. stands for the four components of fitness after 40:

1. F—Flexibility
2. A—Aerobic exercise
3. C—Carry a load
4. E—Equilibrium/balance

F.A.C.E.-ing your future gets an exciting F.A.C.E.-lift in the next chapters.

F—FLEXIBILITY

Our muscles and tendons have a natural tendency to get tighter and stiffer each year we live, and even kids can be "too tight" and get injured. In your after-40 body, this tendency toward tightness and stiffness, and your risk of injury, is even greater. You need to work on flexibility daily.

Chapter 6 teaches you to F.A.C.E your future through flexibility. Since I wrote the first edition, I have become a true believer in foam rolling, Dynamic Stretching and Warm-Up, and Static Stretching in three planes of motion. All of these are included in Chapter 6.

A—AEROBIC EXERCISE

Make it work, then let it rest. Having lots of birthday candles does not mean you cannot be intense. Neither does 20 years of sedentary living. The beauty of using a "speed play" (*fartlek*) approach to aerobic exercise is that—no matter your age or fitness level—you can challenge your body to the next level. Remember, you are in a race with only yourself!

Chapter 7 gives your aerobic exercise a F.A.C.E-lift by teaching you to maximize your cardiovascular fitness (and, therefore, your health) by being intense in your mobility (even if you are stepping off the couch for the first time in years), using progressive overload, managing your exercise volume to maximize your metabolic returns, and learning how the concept of reversibility can ruin your whole game plan.

C—CARRY A LOAD

Step away from the weight machine! In the 29 years I have been taking care of athletes and active people, I have *never* seen anyone actually use his muscles in real life the way we typically train them in the gym. Why is that?

One reason is that in the gym, people are taught to "strengthen" their quadriceps by sitting on a leg press or knee extension machine and lifting the stacks of weight in one plane of motion, without gravity or ground reactive force pushing back against them. In real life, we use our quadriceps in coordination with our butts and cores to squat down to pick up a laundry basket (or a car, as one of my recent patients tried—but that's another story), or we climb stairs with gravity and ground reactive forces pushing back on us. We should train our muscles the way we use them.

Chapter 8 updates the way I train your muscles to carry a load for maximum performance and maximum life. Again, I give you the basics of how to work every muscle group using three planes of motion and gravity or ground reactive forces in the way your body really moves. I also teach you how to design your own program.

Jumping ahead to Chapter 10, however, I go even further for you! What I've learned during the last five years is that people want a very *specific* plan! That's why this edition of *Fitness After 40* includes my nine 20 Minutes to Burn exercise bricks and teaches you how to stack these bricks into a 20-, 40-, or 60-minute workout, depending on how much time you have. The workout is rolled out via a six-week plan to jump-start your mobility.

These workouts have been time-tested by hundreds of active agers, adult-onset exercisers, and true masters athletes—all of whom I have trained via the PRIMA Start program. These workouts are amazing and maximize your body while minimizing injury.

Each of the 20 Minutes to Burn circuits also kills two birds with one stone: You get specific workout instructions, and you can't use the I-don't-have-time excuse. *Everyone* has 20 minutes to burn!

E—EQUILIBRIUM/BALANCE

The final component of building a total body mobility regimen that maximizes your performance and your life is equilibrium/balance.

Right now, I want you to stop reading and stand up. Carefully raise your right foot off the ground and try to balance. If you are still standing after 25 seconds, then close your eyes. There you go looking like the Leaning Tower of Pisa or the London Bridge!

When talking to groups about F.A.C.E.-ing their future, I often stop and ask the audience to stand and balance on one leg. You can imagine what a room full of people toppling over looks like from the stage! It's all fun and games until, in your real life, you fall down and break a bone. As your orthopaedic surgeon and "mobility doc," I can't let this happen to you. That's why Chapter 9 spends time retraining the neuromuscular pathways that control your balance and keeps you on your feet in three planes of motion.

F.A.C.E.-ing your future and being smart works whether you are an AOE (adult-onset exerciser), an OUT-E (once-upon-a-time exerciser), or a true masters athlete trying to maximize your performance and minimize injury.

WHERE ARE YOU NOW?

When I talk to people about their fitness after 40, I divide fitness into four categories as a way to identify where they are starting and where they are going. Look at Table 1 and decide where you are now.

Table 1. Four Categories of Fitness

Who	Current Description	Goals
Elite	Trains daily Competitive High health and fitness reserves	Maximize performance Prevent injury
Fit	Exercises two to three times per week Moderate health and fitness reserves	Maintain and increase performance Prevent injury
Independent (AOEs and OUT-Es)	Lives independently Does not exercise Low health and fitness reserves	Begin to F.A.C.E. a future of physical wealth (i.e., a storage of physical reserves) Move to Fit level
Frail	Performs basic activities of daily living Can't live independently No health reserves	Maintain or improve basic activities of daily living Increase strength and independence

I suspect that few of you reading this book are in the Frail category. If you are, keep reading, because no matter what you are able to do now, your body is always capable of improvement. In a landmark study by Maria Fiatarone, men over 90 years old and living in a nursing home took part in a six-week resistance-training program. Even at this advanced age, they were able to increase their strength and stamina.

You probably fall within the Independent group. If so, you are among the 78 percent of people over 50 who identify keeping active as the most important factor in aging well and yet currently do not invest daily in their physical wealth. A good way to think about this is in terms of storing up health the way we save money. Every day, most of us go to work and make money. We invest some of the money for the future. In the same way, we must invest in our physical futures every day. If you don't exercise daily, you may do all right day to day, but you are not reserving any physical wealth for a rainy day. You are essentially living physical paycheck to paycheck, and when you get sick and need to draw from your saved-up bodily reserves, the bank is empty.

Don't despair! If you are in this category, I am excited for you! You have the most to gain from this book and can make the most significant changes in your health and performance. Your goal is to use the F.A.C.E. principles (coming up in Chapters 6 to 9) to create a plan that works for you. We want to move you up to the next level, being Fit.

If you do purposeful exercise two to three times per week, you are among the 28 percent of people in the United States who are in the Fit category. You are living the dream of all the people who are Independent but not Fit. You will find much valuable information in the following chapters on how to maximize your performance and fitness while taking the necessary steps to remain injury-free.

If you can easily perform your usual workout, it is time to shake it up and challenge yourself. Perhaps instead of just finishing a race, you can challenge those in your age group. If you are plagued by recurrent overuse injuries or aches and pains, I want to help you exercise more smartly so that you can keep yourself out of your doctor's office and on the road.

If you are currently an Elite masters athlete, winning your age division or placing in open competition, I am inspired by you! You are at the same level as the 50-year-old male Senior Olympian (discussed in Chapter 2) whom I witnessed winning the mile sprint in 4:35! I refer to you often when I speak and hold you up as an example of the physical heights we can attain if we are not hindered by the ravages of a sedentary lifestyle. For you, the challenge is to maintain your high level of physical fitness while remaining injury-free. For you, God is in the details.

Carl participated in one of my fitness training groups. I was talking to him about how his training was going and why he was participating in the first place. He observed that, although he had always tried to stay active, as he aged he was continually sidelined by a series of injuries. Start . . . stop . . . start . . . stop. He could never maintain the level of activity he wanted because just as he would ramp up his activity, he would get hurt again. What he liked about my approach, he said, was the focus on being a well-rounded exerciser and learning how to exercise in a smarter way to avoid injury. "Yes!" I practically screamed as I clapped out loud. He got it!

As your orthopaedic surgeon and mobility doc, I promise that F.A.C.E.-ing your future is a smart way to take control of the more than 70 percent of the aging process you control with the decisions you make every day. Now turn the page and let's move to maximize your performance—and your life!

HOMEWORK

Look back at Table 1. Identify which category you are currently in. Review the goals for your current level. Keep them in mind as you make a plan for your future in the coming chapters.

"Those who think they have no time for bodily exercise will sooner or later have to find time for illness."

—Edward Stanley, British statesman

CHAPTER **SIX** 6

F—Flexibility

It may be hard to imagine, but even kids can be "too tight" and get injured as a result. And, with each year we live, muscles and tendons have a natural tendency to get tighter and stiffer. This means your after-40 body runs a greater risk of injury than it used to, which is why you need to work on flexibility daily.

You and I know that remaining flexible is good for us. Focusing on flexibility, however, is my least favorite part of my fitness regimen, and you may feel the same way. Flexibility is easy to ignore, and many active people *do* ignore it. The truth is that, by and large, the active agers and athletes who come into my office with repetitive injuries are stiff as boards! Their hamstrings, their calves, their shoulders, and their backs are all stiff. This perpetual tightness often leads to injury and frustration. These people are not limited by the number of years they have lived but by the length of their muscles. It doesn't have to be this way! You grew these muscles, and you can make them perform for you in just 15 minutes per day.

Flexibility is the ability of muscle to lengthen and allow your joints to move through a full range of motion. Maintaining muscle flexibility increases athletic performance, improves running economy (decreased energy expenditure at a given speed), prevents injury, decreases soreness, and hastens rehabilitation following injury. In their relaxed state, muscles (and the tendons that attach them to your bones) are "crinkled" up. (This is literally the scientific term for their accordion-like resting state.) When they are in a chronically shortened state, muscles and tendons prevent our joints from moving through their full range of motion, which changes the way we walk, our posture, and, among other things, our golf swing (heaven forbid). Not only this, but stiff muscles and tendons are like the old, dried-out rubber bands you find in the back of your desk drawer. One pull and these brittle old bands "pop" and sideline us with injury.

I have an elite masters sprinter named Ron who trains at our performance center. He is incredibly driven and works with high intensity to explode down the track. I first saw Ron because he was experiencing pain in his hamstrings (the muscles in the back of the thighs responsible for powerful knee flexion). When I assessed him, I found that his hamstrings were tight like guitar strings. I would almost "twang" them with my finger as I flexed his hip and tried to straighten his leg into the air. This is a scary situation for any sprinter, but especially for a masters sprinter whose muscles and tendons are aging. Daily stretching was not a part of Ron's workout regimen. We talked for a long time about flexibility and the priority it should be for him. He was not F.A.C.E.-ing his competitive future; rather, he had continued to do the types of workouts he had done since his twenties. Unfortunately, he could not undo the years of progressive hamstring tightening overnight, and he ultimately injured his hamstring. He has been carefully rehabilitated back to competitive form, but paying attention to flexibility in the first place would have saved him a lot of pain and improved his sprinting.

Here is another example of what I'm talking about. You have all seen elderly people walking around with bent knees all stooped over. While there can be many reasons for this, one big reason people start walking with bent knees is shortening of the hamstrings. As previously said, the hamstrings are the large muscles in the back of your leg. They connect your pelvis to your lower leg. Hamstrings act as the rubber band that flexes your knee during walking or, more powerfully, during exercise. After years in a crinkled state, muscles like hamstrings get shorter. The thigh bone (femur), however, does not get shorter, so the only way you can make the distance between the pelvis and lower leg shorter is to bend your knees. Well, you can't walk with bent knees and straight hips, so to compensate, you bend your hips forward. Before you know it, you are walking around with a stooped gait—looking old.

Flexibility is essential in preventing all kinds of injuries, but tendinitis (discussed in Chapter 2) in particular. Prevention of tendinitis requires stretching the muscle on a regular basis, which allows less pulling and traction on the tendon's attachment to the bone. When tendinitis does occur, it is important to treat it immediately and prevent it from reaching the more severe stage, called tendonosis. Even if you have not reached for your toes in years, it is not too late to start stretching and regaining your flexibility.

Since I wrote the first edition, foam rolling, Dynamic Stretching and Warm-Up, and Static Stretching in three planes of motion have become extremely important in my beliefs about exercise. The rest of this chapter teaches you these three components of flexibility for maximizing your performance—on the road and in life.

THE FACTS ON FLEXIBILITY

Here are the down-and-dirty, scientifically proven facts for regaining and maintaining your flexibility. First, you must stretch every day. Yes, *every* day! When I say this to my patients, I often see a look in their eyes that says, "When am I going to fit this in?" To which I reply, "I mean it. Get out of bed, hop in the shower, get out, stretch for 15 minutes, and then get on with your day."

One amazing way to gently work on your tight problem areas is by using a foam roller. This firm tube of foam is a godsend to my patients. Although foam rolling initially hurts, as your tight muscles and tendons lengthen via an active tissue release, it "hurts so good." Foam rolling first thing in the morning (after a hot shower) leaves you limber for the day.

On the following pages I outline foam rolling techniques, six Dynamic Stretching and Warm-Up exercises, and 11 Static Stretching exercises you should pay attention to daily. You can accomplish most of this in only 15 minutes a day—as the first 30-second-long slow stretch in each exercise is the most important rep. (The additional reps I describe are a bonus.)

If morning doesn't work for you to work on your flexibility, take 45 minutes to eat lunch instead of an hour and use the other 15 to stretch. (Stretching usually does not make people break a sweat, so there's no need to change into workout clothes midday to do this.) Alternatively, you can stretch in the evening while you watch TV. Stretching does not have to be done all at once either. You can break the stretching regimen up over the course of the day and do one body part at a time.

I currently teach people to regain maximum muscle and tendon flexibility via foam rolling, Dynamic Stretching, and Static Stretching. Foam rolling can loosen known problem areas on your entire body prior to aerobic exercise. Dynamic Stretching and Warm-Up is also performed prior to aerobic exercise or, if performed intensely enough, can actually also serve as the aerobic portion of your exercise. Static Stretching—holding your stretch for 30 to 60 seconds without moving—is reserved for when you are warmed up.

FOAM ROLLING

"Go buy a foam roller." I commonly say these words to most of my athletes of all ages and skill levels. Foam rolling is a marvelous way to stretch your tight tendons and muscles and work out your problem areas before activity (or at any time at all). Foam rolling on the living room floor while watching the news or your favorite show is a great way for you to maximize your body and your brain. (Photos 1 through 5 show the use of a foam roller on different parts of the body.)

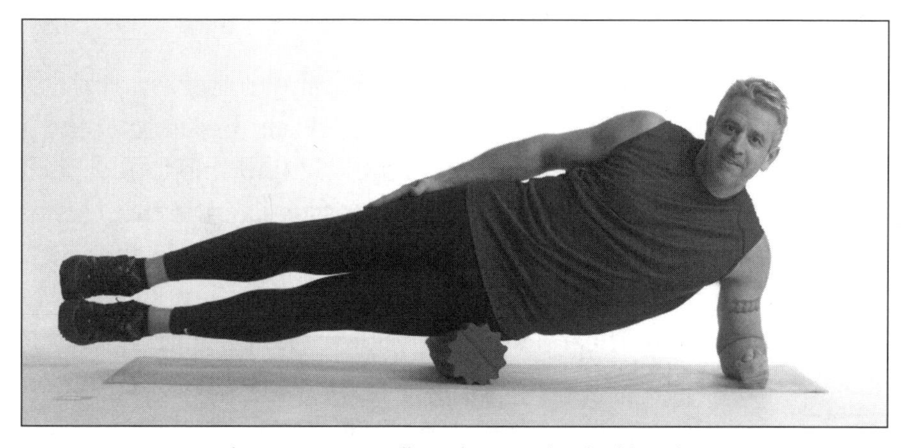

Photo 1. Foam rolling the ITB (iliotibial band).

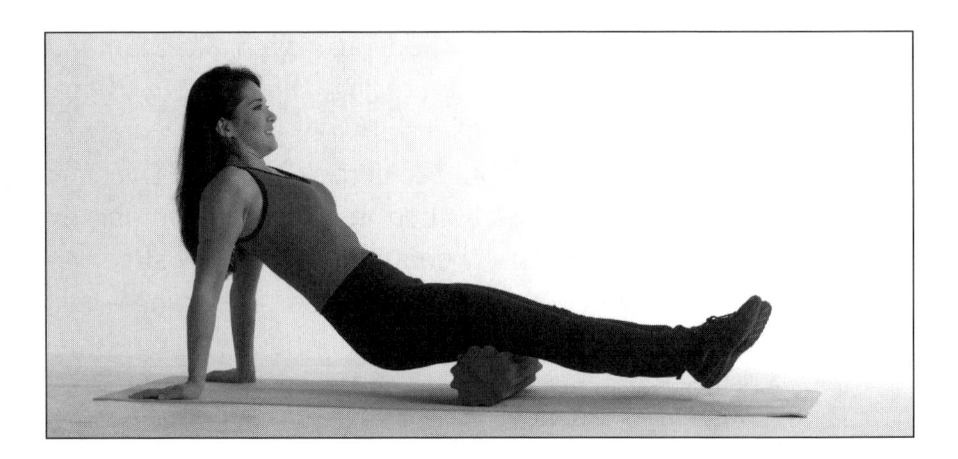

Photo 2. Foam rolling the hamstrings.

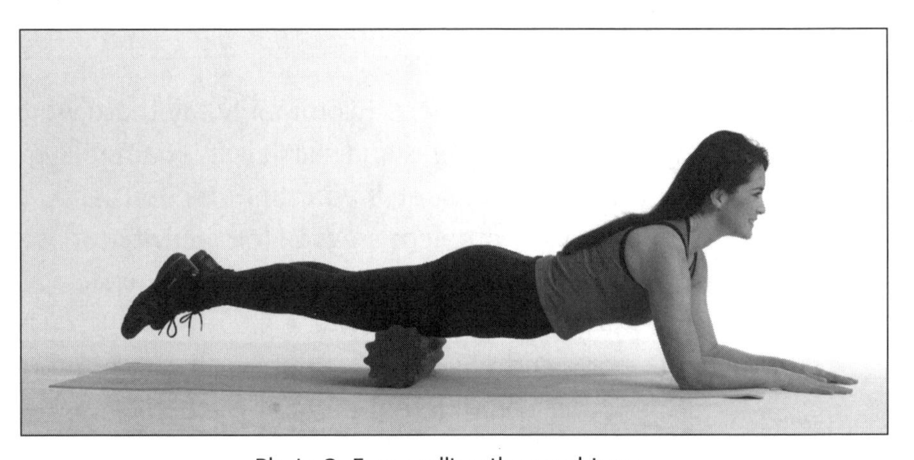

Photo 3. Foam rolling the quadriceps.

Essentially, the log of hard foam serves as a rolling pin to break up small adhesions and scar tissue, thereby increasing blood flow to problem areas. I find this tool especially good for stretching hard-to-stretch tissue like the muscles of the legs and the iliotibial band (ITB), which runs down the side of your legs from hip to knee. Nothing could be simpler than lying on a foam roller and using your upper body to pull yourself slowly back and forth across the roller. The most common areas to foam roll are the ITBs, quadriceps, hamstrings, adductors, buttocks, and calves.

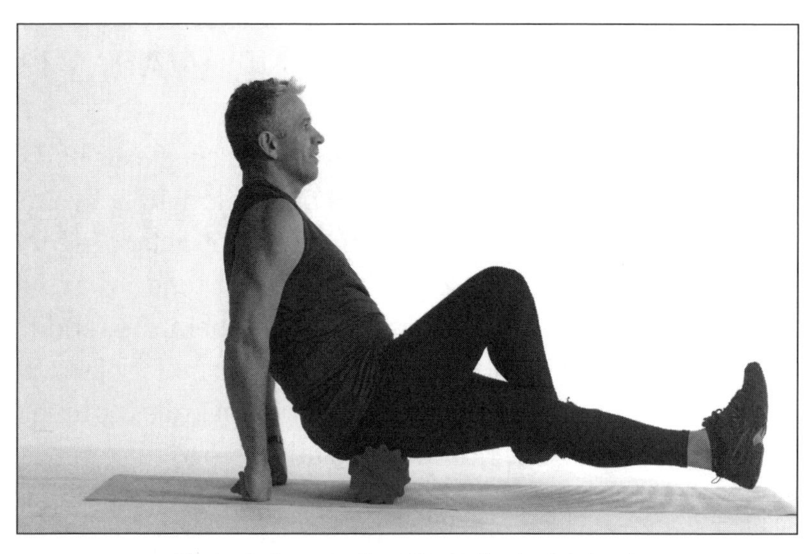

Photo 4. Foam rolling the buttocks (gluteus).

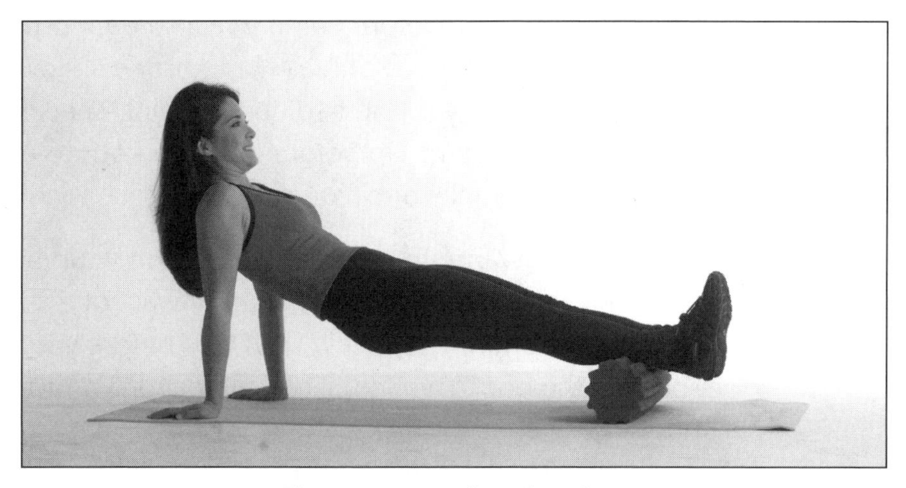

Photo 5. Foam rolling the calves.

1. Place the foam roller directly under the muscle group to be rolled.
2. Place your full body weight on the roller.
3. Pull your body back and forth slowly over the roller using your upper body.
4. Roll five times over each muscle group.

DYNAMIC STRETCHING AND WARM-UP

Warming up is more than just raising your body temperature. A good warm-up increases blood flow to active muscles, allows for efficient functionality of both contracting (agonist) and relaxing (antagoist) muscles, loosens tight tendons and muscle resistance to motion, increases muscle temperature (and therefore oxygen delivery), and jump-starts muscle metabolism for action. In short, a good warm-up allows *you*—regardless of whether you are an AOE, OUT-E, or masters athlete—to maximize the efficacy of your workout, in addition to possibly reducing injury.

Like many life-long runners who developed habits as a kid, I spent years wasting the first couple of miles of every workout getting warmed up before I hit my real stride. I usually dreaded that period from "shoes on" to "in the zone." Now, older and wiser, I teach all my runners to do a running-specific Dynamic Stretching and Warm-Up before each workout to minimize injury and make every mile or circuit count.

You must warm up before taking off on your exercise adventure. This can take the form of an easy walk or a slow jog before a run or, for swimmers, a few slow laps before you turn up the speed in the pool. Dynamic Stretching and Warm-Ups—warm-ups where you are moving and stretching instead of just standing in one place—are fun and get the heart pumping and the muscles filled with blood. You go from relatively "cold" to "warm" and ready to go.

A great way to get the most out of your Dynamic Stretching and Warm-Up is to jog/walk for 20–30 yards (or do another planned aerobic activity, such as stair climbing, bike riding, swimming, and so forth) between each exercise set. This is the impulse behind the *fartlek* concept, which we discuss at length in Chapter 7. Alternatively, Dynamic Stretching and Warm-Ups can in and of themselves serve as a workout to improve strength, power, and agility. With dynamic movements, your muscles are lengthened and then a contraction occurs in the lengthened position, providing more functional range of motion. Traditional Static Stretching (discussed later in this chapter) should be reserved for when you are already warmed up.

Dynamic Stretching and Warm-Ups can be sport-specific and designed to mobilize the movement patterns, muscles, joints, and planes of motion needed for a particular activity. However, the following stretches can be performed before any kind of exercise.

Hip Circle

This exercise warms up the large muscles in the front and back of your midsection and buttocks.

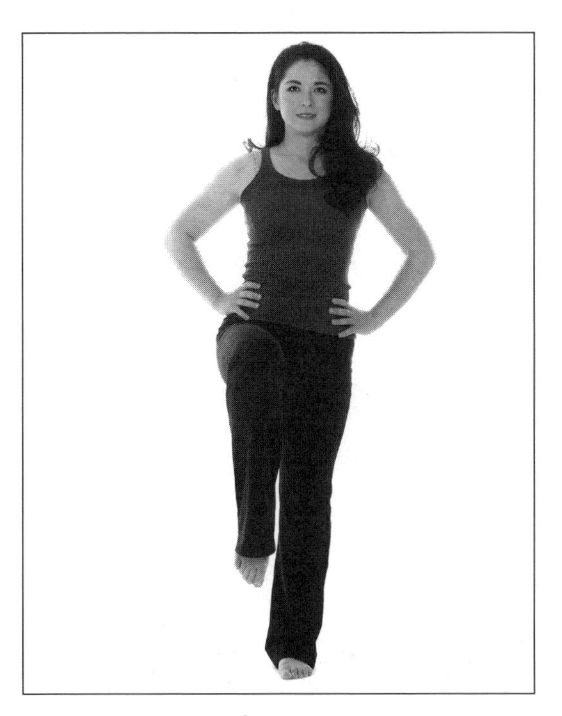

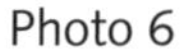

Photo 6

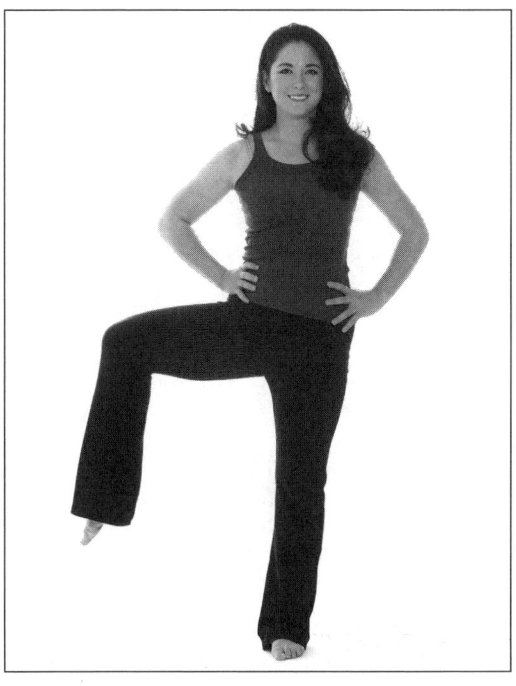

Photo 7

1. Begin with your hands on your hips and your feet together.
2. Bend one leg up in front of the body at the hip (as shown in Photo 6) and rotate it up to the side (as shown in Photo 7), then lower it.
3. Reverse the movement by bending the same leg up at the hip to the side and rotating it forward before lowering it.
4. Repeat Steps 1–3 10 times.
5. Perform with the opposite leg.

Lunge

This exercise not only warms up your hips and buttocks but also stretches your hip flexor muscles.

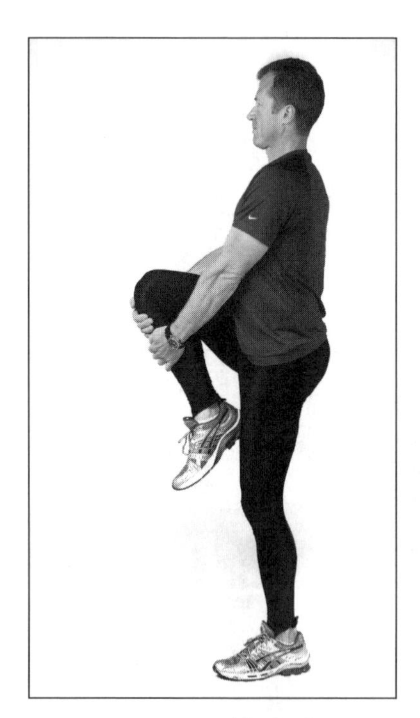

Photo 8

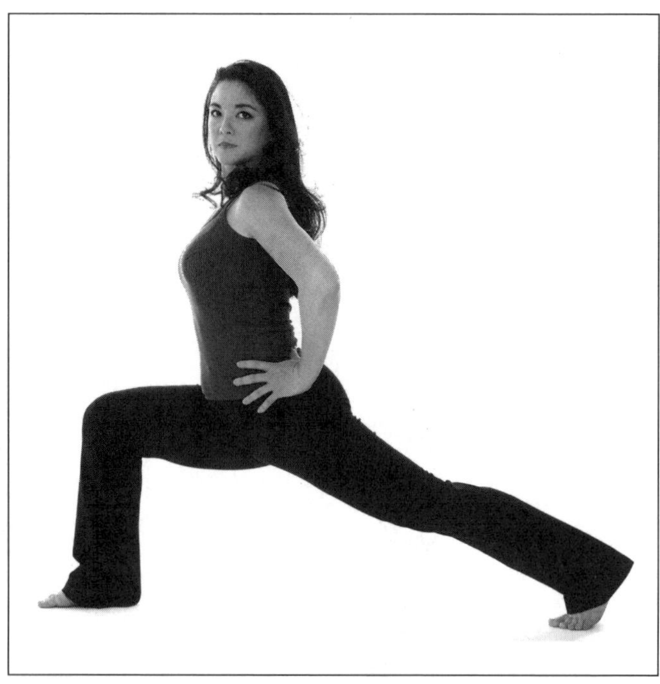

Photo 9

1. Stand with your feet together.
2. Hug one of your knees to your chest (as shown in Photo 8) and then release your leg.
3. Lunge onto that knee while trying to keep your knee above your ankle and not in front of it (as shown in Photo 9).
4. Bring your back leg forward until you are standing again.
5. Repeat Steps 1–4 10 times with the same leg, and progress forward.
6. Perform with the opposite leg.

Activator

This exercise, which is harder than it looks, warms up your legs while giving a good stretch to the hamstrings and calf muscles that run down the backs of your legs.

1. Begin in a push-up position (as shown in Photo 10).
2. Slowly walk your legs toward your hands (as shown in Photo 11). Your heels may be off the floor.
3. Continue walking forward until the pull in the back of your legs is uncomfortable.
4. At this point, slowly walk your arms forward with your feet still (as shown in Photo 12), until you are back in the push-up position.
5. Repeat Steps 1–4 five to 10 times.

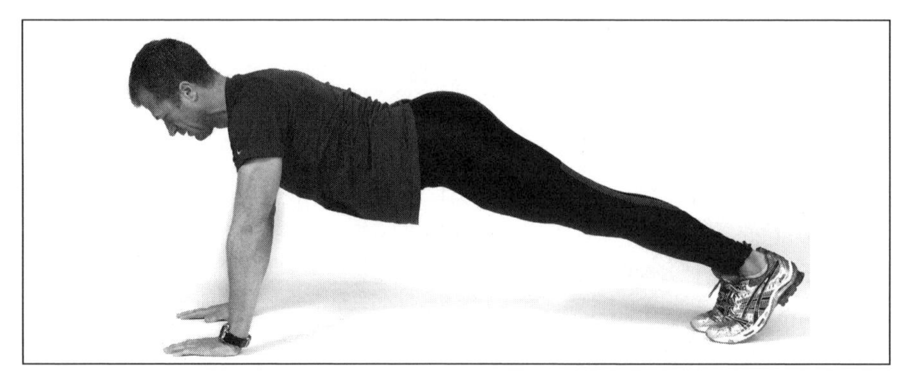

Photo 10

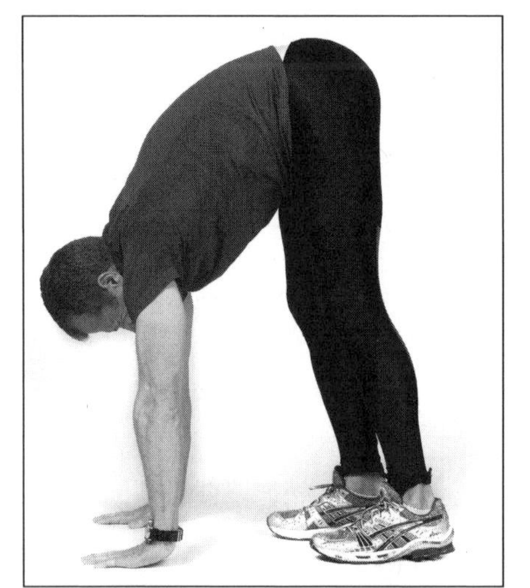

Photo 11. Walk legs forward.

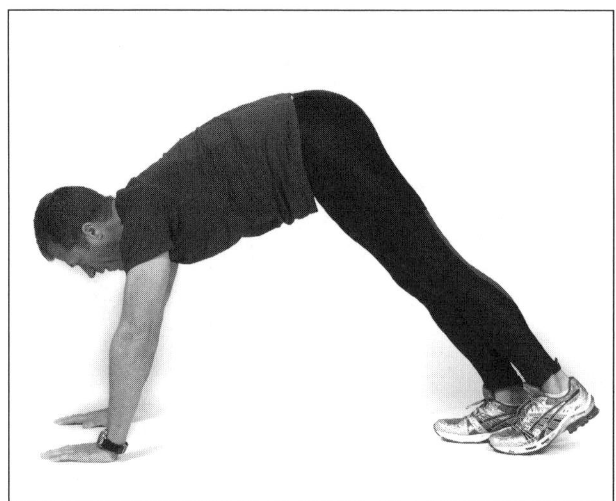

Photo 12. Walk arms forward.

Toe and Heel Walk

Walking on your toes gives your calves, in the back of your lower legs, a good warm-up. Walking on your heels warms up the front portion of your legs as well as warms up your ankles. If your legs start to ache while doing either of these walks, you should stop.

1. Walk on your toes with your toes pointed straight ahead for about 20 meters (a meter is about a yard), getting as high up on your toes as you possibly can. Your legs should be relatively straight as you do this, and you should—at least initially—take fairly small steps.
2. Switch to walking on your toes with your feet rotated out for 20 meters.
3. Do the same with your toes pointed in for 20 meters.
4. Repeat Steps 1–3 while walking on your heels.

Skip

Did you think skipping was just for kids? It's not. It's a good way for you to warm up. Skipping can also be used to vary your runs. Sometimes when I am tired and bored during a marathon, I switch to skipping for a few hundred meters to break it up a bit.

1. Skip for 20 meters, landing on your mid-foot area with each contact with the ground, and with your toes pointed straight ahead.
2. Try skipping for 20 meters by flexing your knees up high and taking longer than normal strides.

Rhythm Bounding

Bounding is just what it sounds like. You spring up into the air with each step you take. It looks like you are jogging with high knees in slow motion.

1. On a springy surface, such as a rubber track or grass field, jog with short springy steps while landing on your mid-foot area, not on your toes.

2. Spring upward once after each impact. This warms up your ankles and legs by making them act like coiled springs. You move forward and upward with each step.

STATIC STRETCHING

Changes in flexibility are dependent on the frequency and duration of stretching. For people younger than 65, maximum benefit from Static Stretching is achieved with a slow muscle stretch until the muscle feels tight but doesn't hurt. (Slow stretching lengthens muscle fibers without causing tears and damage. This is important since muscle tears often heal with scars, which are very stiff.) Once you reach this place, hold the stretch for 30 seconds without bouncing. While any amount of stretching is better than nothing, less than 30 seconds is less effective. After 30 seconds, rest for 10 seconds and then repeat the stretch for a maximum of four repetitions. Remember that the most benefit comes from the first long-slow 30-second rep. It is okay to do only one rep if time is an issue. Note: If you are under 65, you do not achieve any additional benefit by holding the stretch for more than 30 seconds or doing more than four reps.

The guidelines (and benefits) change slightly for people who are 65 and older. Then, you need to hold the stretch for 60 seconds. You should also do four reps.

Perform each set of stretches *once* a day. If you get tight again during the course of the day, you can repeat as necessary (since, once stretched, it is unfortunately natural for your body not to stay that way). Some people are in the habit of doing 20 to 30 repetitions at a time. However, this is unnecessary; no added benefit has been found from doing more than one set per day for each muscle group.

It takes about six weeks of consistent stretching to see good results, and then you must maintain your muscle length by continuing daily stretches. Studies have found that if you stretch for six weeks and then take four weeks off, you will return to baseline as if you had never put in the effort. The good news is that by starting over, you can regain your flexibility again . . . after six weeks.

In summary:

- If you are younger than 65, you should hold each stretch 30 seconds and do four repetitions once a day.
- If are 65 or older, you should hold each stretch 60 seconds and do four repetitions once a day.

This means that it takes only about two minutes to stretch each muscle group and about 15 to 20 minutes for the whole body. Also, while it seems correct intuitively, stretching one side does not increase the flexibility of the other side. You need to stretch both sides.

The exercises that appear on the following pages present a simple and effective general plan for daily stretching.

NECK, UPPER BACK, AND CHEST

Many of us carry our stress and daily tension in the upper back and in one of the muscles (called the trapezius) that connects the shoulder blade to the spine. The trapezius muscle can knot up and become so tight that it causes headaches in the back and sides of the head. The following stretches and range-of-motion exercises should be performed daily and any time you begin to feel tightness in your neck and upper back.

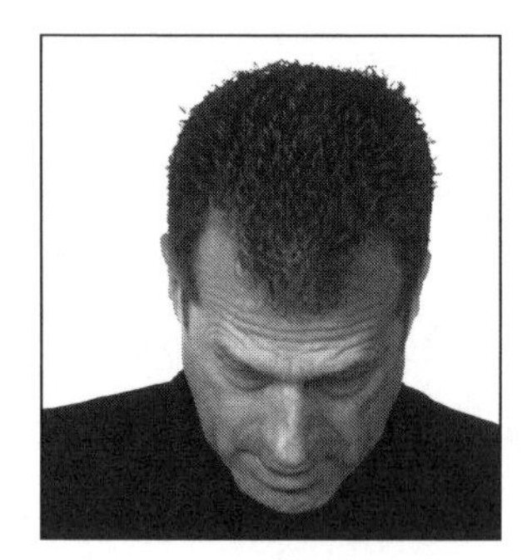

Photo 13

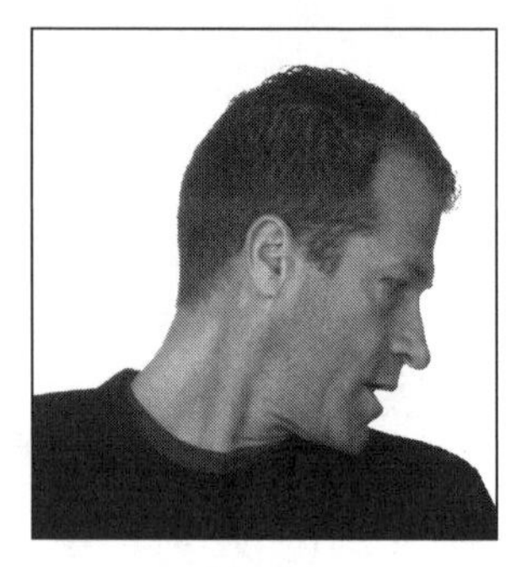

Photo 14

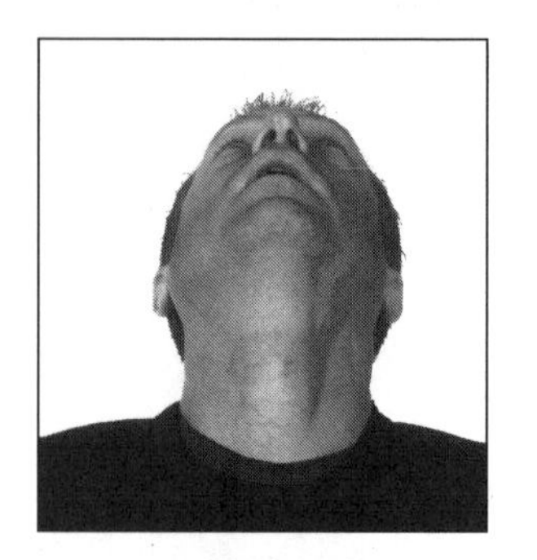

Photo 15

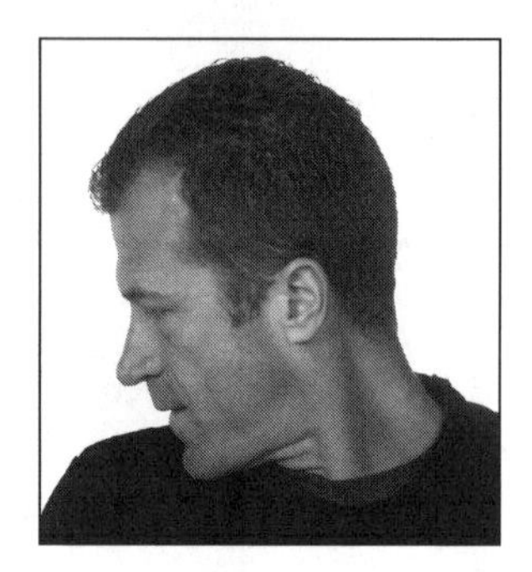

Photo 16

Neck Range of Motion

This exercise should be performed in a slow, continuous arc, so that you are moving your chin from front to side to back to side.

1. Begin in a seated position.
2. Leading with your chin, bend your neck forward so that your chin moves toward your chest (as shown in Photo 13). You will feel a stretch down the back of your neck and across your upper shoulders.
3. Next, turn your chin toward your left shoulder and try to touch your shoulder with your chin (as shown in Photo 14). If you cannot reach your shoulder, don't worry. Don't raise your shoulder to meet your chin.
4. Extend your neck back so that your chin is facing the ceiling (as shown in Photo 15). You may feel pressure in the back of your neck and shoulder blades.
5. Finally, turn your chin toward your right shoulder (as shown in Photo 16). Again, do not raise your shoulder to meet your chin.
6. Return to the starting point.
7. Repeat Steps 2–6 four times. You may hear some crunching in your neck as your head moves on your spine. Painless crunching is fine. However, if pain shoots down your arms or your hands become numb when doing this exercise, stop and make an appointment with your orthopaedic surgeon to make sure your nerves are not being pinched.

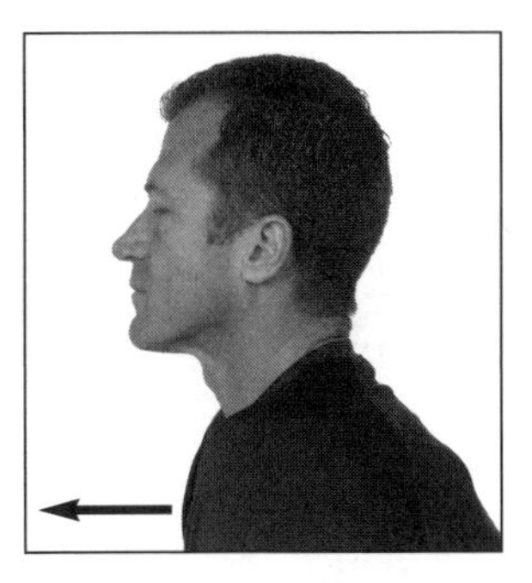

Photo 17. Shoulders move forward.

Shoulder Roll

Many of us sit hunched over a desk all day. We allow our shoulders to slide forward and our back muscles between our shoulder blades to become weak and lax. This eventually leads to a rounded shoulder posture, gives us upper backaches, and makes us look shorter. Do the following exercise at least once a day and any time you sense that you are sliding back into a slumped shoulder posture.

1. In a seated position, let your shoulders relax.
2. Flex your chest (pectoralis) muscles by bringing your shoulders forward (as shown in Photo 17).
3. In a continuous motion, flex your trapezius muscles (between your neck and shoulders) by raising your shoulders up (as shown in Photo 18).
4. Finally, squeeze the muscles between your shoulder blades and bring your shoulders back and down (as shown in Photos 19 and 20).
5. Repeat Steps 2–4 four times, and then try to maintain this upright posture throughout the day.

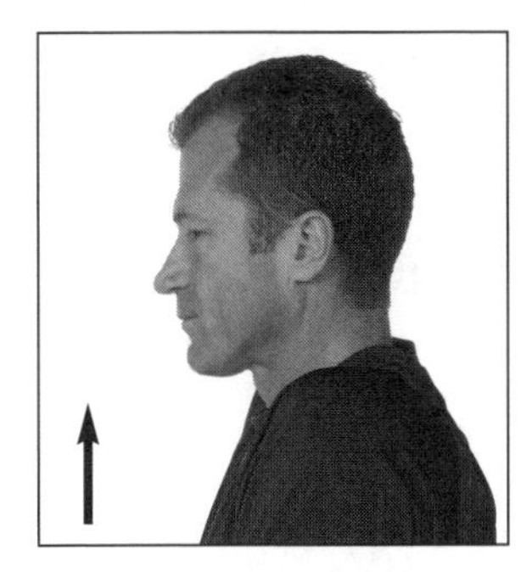

Photo 18. Shoulders move up.

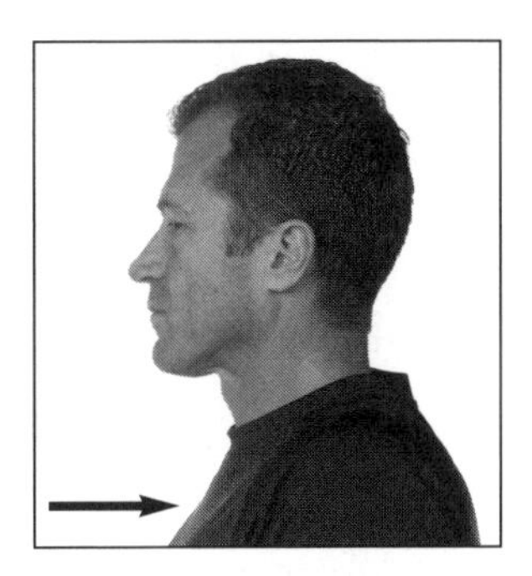

Photo 19. Shoulders move back.

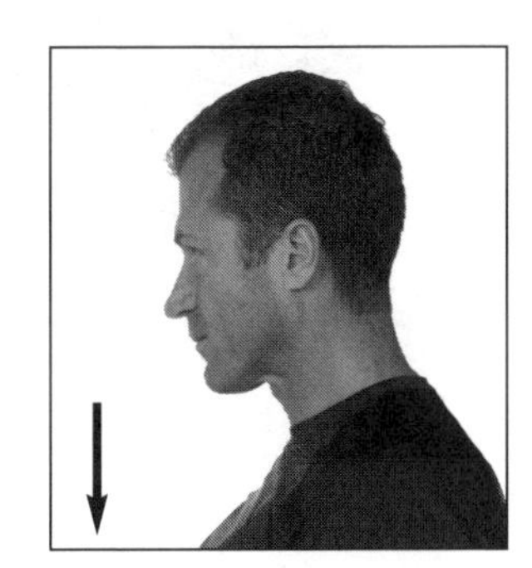

Photo 20. Shoulders move down.

When doing this exercise, keep your upper back muscles contracted and your shoulders back. Your chest should be raised with your shoulders in this position. You may notice that you are sitting higher in your chair, and it should feel great. You may even want to stand sideways in front of a mirror and notice your improved posture!

As I was sitting here writing and performing this range-of-motion exercise, my right shoulder blade popped. Popping is fine unless it is painful or causes mechanical-type locking. Popping in any joint that is not painful usually represents simple movement of tendons or ligaments across the bones.

Seated Trapezius Stretch

Now that your shoulders are back and your upper back is straight, stretch your trapezius muscle with this exercise.

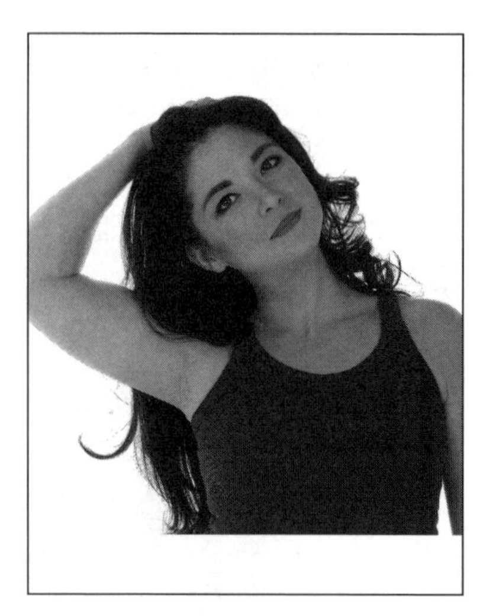

Photo 21

1. In a seated position, tilt your head toward your right shoulder. (You can also do this entire stretch while standing.)
2. Place your right hand over the top of your head and gently pull it down toward the right (as shown in Photo 21). You will feel a stretch in your left trapezius, and if you touch the left side of your neck with your left hand, you will feel the tight muscle being stretched. Hold this stretch for 30 seconds and then relax. Repeat this stretch four times, remembering to breathe.
3. Now tilt your head toward your left shoulder. Place your left hand over the top of your head and gently pull down to stretch your right trapezius muscle. Again, hold

this stretch for 30 seconds and then relax. Repeat four times.

You may want to vary this routine by transitioning directly from a single Shoulder Roll (the previous exercise) to a right and then left Trapezius Stretch, and then repeating the three stretches again in that sequence four additional times.

Chest Stretch

You are going to hear me say this many times: *The key to the back is the front!* Usually, I say this in relation to the lower back and core, but even in the upper back and shoulders, we cannot forget to stretch our chest muscles. People who work out a lot usually focus on their pectoralis muscles and building a big chest. (Who can blame them? It looks great.) The problem is that a chest that is tight and contracted only adds to the posture

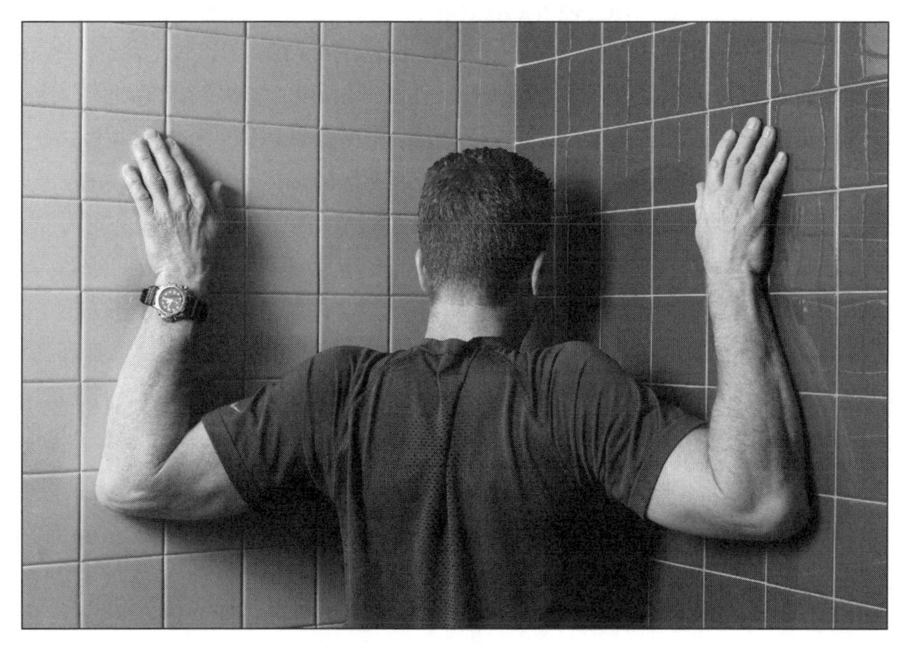

Photo 22

problems and back tension we were working on in the previous three exercises. So now, let's stretch our chests.

1. Find a corner or doorway to stand in.
2. Raise your arms to shoulder height and bend your elbows 90 degrees so that your palms are against the wall and your fingertips are facing the ceiling.
3. Place your feet shoulder-width apart and lean forward (as shown in Photo 22). You should feel a stretch across your chest. If you do not, then step back another step and lean forward again. Hold this position for 30 seconds, relax, and repeat four times.

SHOULDERS AND ARMS

Our shoulders and arms are the mainstay of our daily productivity. We do not realize how much we rely on them until even a small pain sidelines us or wakes us from sleep. The following stretches (coupled with the exercises in "Fitness to Go: Your Shoulders and Arms" in Chapter 8) will take you a long way toward peak shoulder and arm performance.

Shoulder Stretch

We usually do a good job maintaining shoulder motion to the front and sides simply through normal daily use. However, we do not do as good a job at keeping the back of our shoulders and rotator cuff (the four small muscles that keep our shoulder joint together) well stretched unless we specifically focus on it. Keeping the back part of the shoulder flexible helps the rotator

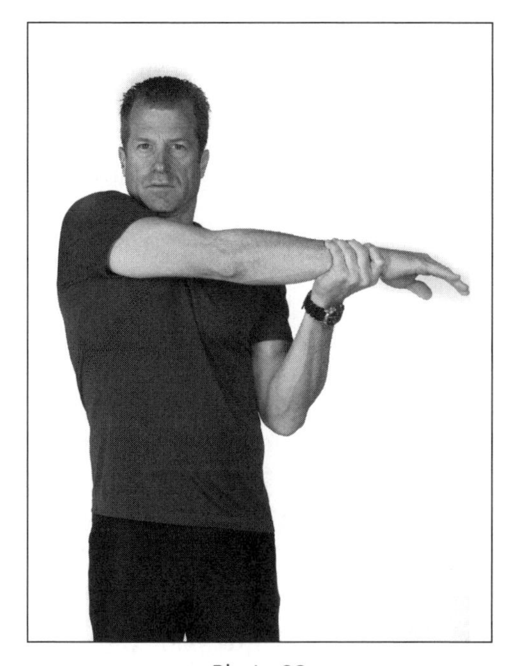

Photo 23

cuff maintain shoulder stability. This is true for regular people like you and me as well as elite athletes such as baseball pitchers. Flexibility in the back of the shoulder is key to keeping your arm well centered in your shoulder socket.

1. Stand with your feet shoulder-width apart.
2. Raise your right arm up to shoulder height and move it across the front of your body.
3. With your left arm, pull the right arm as close to your chest as possible (as shown in Photo 23) and hold it for 30 seconds. You should feel the stretch across the back of your shoulder. Then relax.
4. Repeat Steps 2–3 four times, then switch to the left arm.

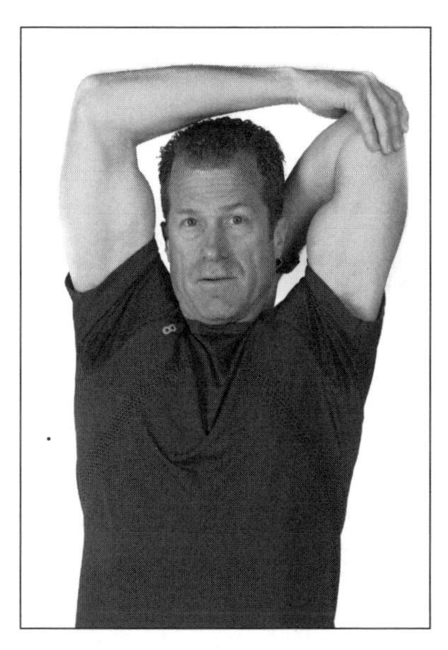

Photo 24

Triceps Stretch

This exercise keeps your triceps (the muscle on the back of the upper arm) stretched.

1. With your feet shoulder-width apart, raise your left arm up, then bend your elbow so your hand falls behind your back.
2. Raise your right arm and bend your elbow so that your right hand is grasping your left elbow (as shown in Photo 24).

3. Gently pull on your left elbow. You will feel a great stretch in the back of your left arm and upper shoulder. Hold this position for 30 seconds, then relax.
4. Repeat Steps 1–3 four times, then switch to the right side. Remember to breathe while you do this. (It feels great!)

LOWER BACK

"Oh, my aching back!" This complaint is shared by so many people. But what is the key to your back? Say it with me: *The key to my back is my front*. In "Fitness to Go: Your Lower Back and Core" in Chapter 8, you will learn exercises that revitalize the strength of these areas. Your core muscles are your natural weight belt. To find them, put your hand on your waist, then suck in your belly button toward your spine. Did you feel the muscles under your skin get tight? These are your core muscles. They run obliquely from your spine to the front of your body. If you were not able to feel these muscles, try bearing down like you are going to the bathroom. You should be able to feel them now. Everything we do begins with our core muscles. These are the top of the exercise food chain as far as I'm concerned.

Until we get to Chapter 8, though, what can you do now if your back is killing you? Lower back stretches will help.

Lower Back Stretch

Multiple layers of paraspinal muscles and oblique core muscles support your upright posture. These muscles originate on or near your spine and will be stretched and relaxed with this exercise.

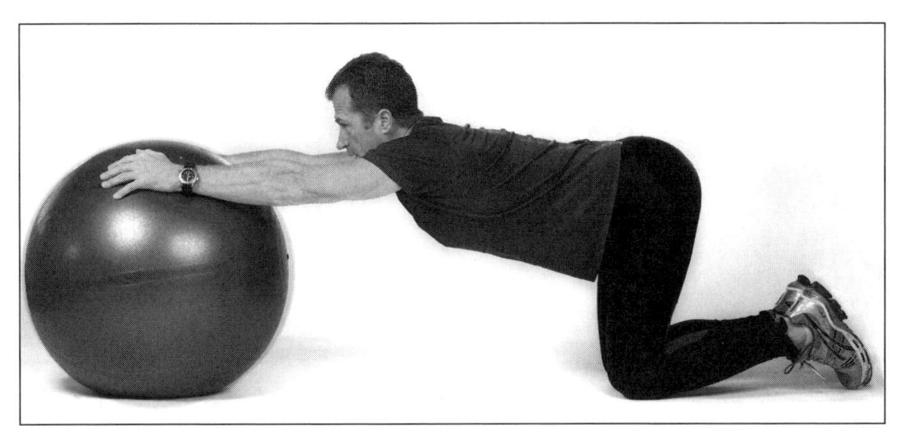

Photo 25

1. Begin on your knees.
2. Place your hands in front of you on an exercise ball or the seat of a chair.
3. While keeping your back flat, reach forward with your arms (as shown in Photo 25) and lower your buttocks to your feet. You will feel a stretch along the sides of your back.
4. Hold for 30 seconds, while breathing, then relax.

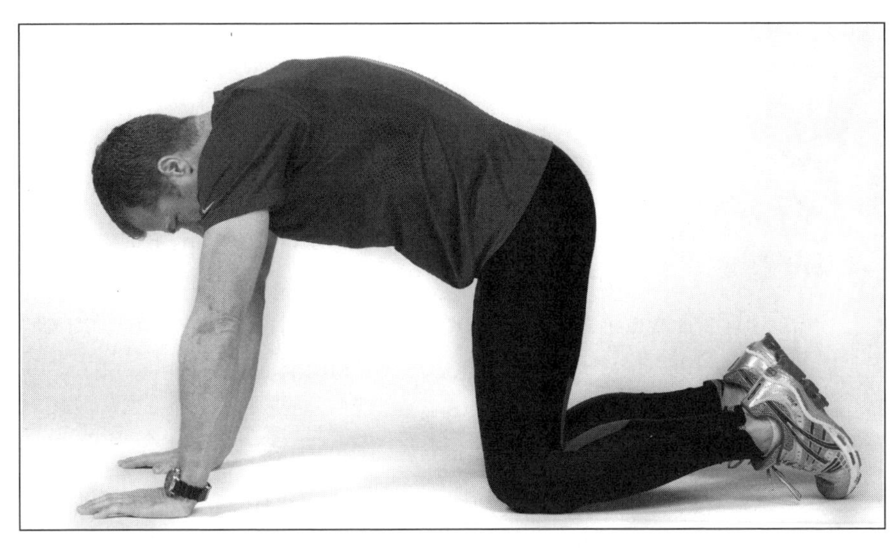

Photo 26

5. Repeat Steps 2–4 four times. Next, place your hands shoulder-width apart on the ground. It will look like you are crawling.
6. Gently arch your back toward the ceiling and tuck your buttocks in (as shown in Photo 26). Hold for 30 seconds, then relax.
7. Repeat Step 6 four times.
8. After the last arch, lower your buttocks to your heels with your arms stretched out front and let your back relax.

HIPS AND LEGS

There are many ways to accomplish a stretch. You may have learned to stretch your legs in different ways as you worked with different coaches. The following hip and leg stretches will give you a general approach to the lower body. Remember, as always, to hold each stretch for 30 seconds, repeat four times, and never bounce. If you find you are having difficulty balancing during these stretches, read Chapter 9 on regaining your equilibrium, and perform these stretches with something nearby to hold on to.

Hip Flexor Stretch in Three Planes

The hip flexors include two muscles that join into one tendon to flex your hips, called the iliopsoas. All muscles in your body move in three planes of motion, and this stretch elongates the hip flexors in all three planes.

1. Stand with your feet together.
2. Step forward with your right leg into a lunge position. Bring your left knee toward the ground while keeping your right knee aligned above your ankle and your hips forward. At this

point, you will be in a lunge position (as shown in Photo 9 earlier in this chapter).

3. Raise both of your arms above your head. You should feel a gentle stretch in the front of your back leg. Hold this position for 30 seconds, then lower your arms.
4. Then, lean your trunk toward your right leg and raise your left arm over your head. Hold this position for 30 seconds, then lower your arm.
5. Finally, raise your left arm above your body and twist your trunk so your left elbow passes to the right of your right knee. This opens up the left side of your body. Hold this position for 30 seconds, then lower your arm.
6. Switch legs and repeat Steps 2–5.
7. Repeat the rotations, right and left, four times.

Holding your legs in a lunge like this for 90 seconds (30 seconds in each position) may initially be too much for you. That is fine. Work up to it.

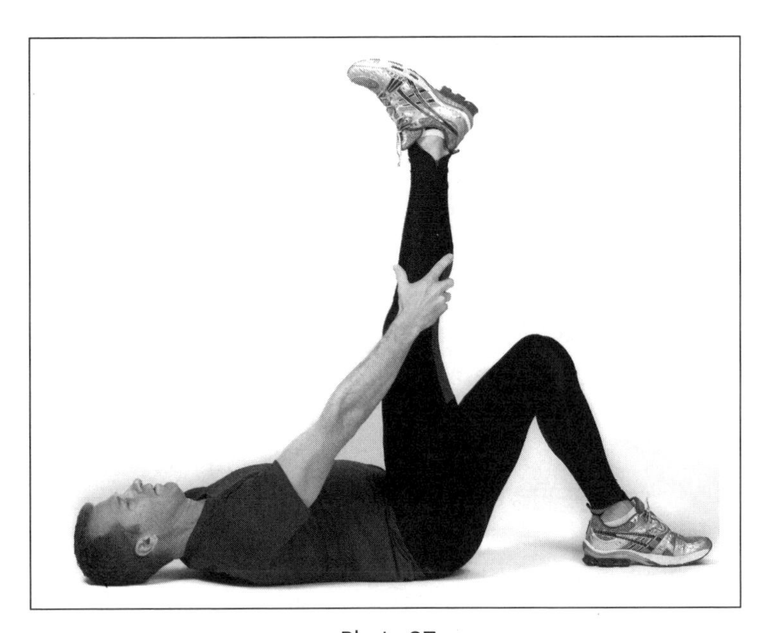

Photo 27

Hamstring Stretch

Hamstrings are powerful muscles that cross the hip joint as well as the knee joint, driving hip extension and knee flexion. They are especially vulnerable to injury whenever our explosive athletic demands overcome their flexibility. Therefore, regardless of your age, it is critical to maintain the flexibility of your hamstrings.

The Hamstring Stretch can be performed lying on the ground as shown in Photo 27 or can be as simple as raising your heel up on a stool or chair and leaning forward. I do my personal favorite variation after I run. While still out in the park or on the sidewalk, I place my feet a little more than shoulder-width apart and lean forward with a straight back from the waist. With my knees straight, I place my palms on the ground, which gives me a great stretch in the back of my legs. To increase the stretch, all I have to do is move my feet closer together until, when I'm really flexible, my feet are together and my palms are on the ground.

Years ago, when I was a ballet dancer, I loved to do the Hamstring Stretch in the following way:

1. Lie down with the small of your back against the floor.
2. Bend your left knee to 90 degrees to stabilize your hips.
3. Slowly raise your right leg off the ground with the knee as straight as possible. Your right hip should not rise off the floor and the motion should be coming only from your hip. As your foot approaches vertical, you will feel a stretch in the back of your leg.

4. Hold your leg in this raised position for 30 seconds (as shown in Photo 27). As you become more flexible, your foot and knee will come past vertical and get closer to your chest and ear. (It's true. That is why I loved this stretch as a dancer.)

5. Relax your knee and then repeat Steps 2–4 four times before switching to the left leg.

You can modify this exercise by placing a towel around the sole of your shoe and, keeping your leg straight, pulling your leg toward your chest.

Quadriceps Stretch

If you were in my office with knee pain, you would hear me say, "The quads are the key to the knees!" The quadriceps—a giant set of four muscles (thus the name quads) in the front of the legs—are powerful knee protectors. They cross two joints—the hip and knee—and are responsible for some hip flexion and all knee extension. They also are key in absorbing the shock of our body weight across the knee and for keeping our kneecaps aligned down the center of the knee. Learn this stretch and pay special attention to the "Fitness to Go: Your Butt, Quads, and Knees" section in Chapter 8.

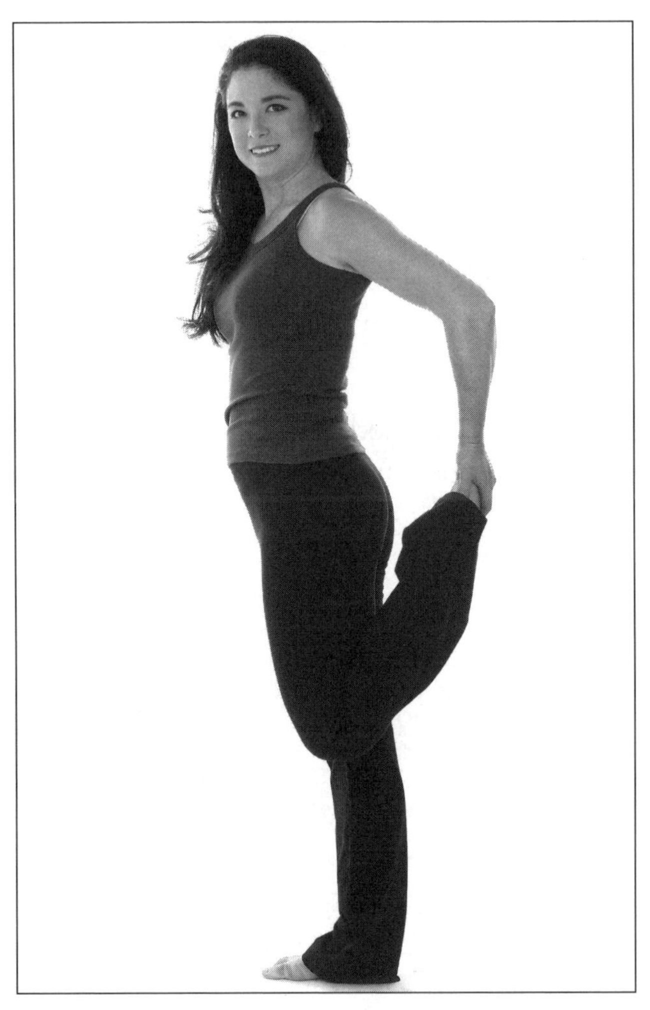

Photo 28

1. Stand with your feet together and hips straight.
2. Bend your left knee and take the front of your left foot in your left hand. If you have trouble with your balance, stand near a chair and steady yourself with your right hand.
3. Keeping your knees even (i.e., do not let your left knee swing forward), pull your left leg back (as shown in Photo 28). You will feel a stretch in the front of your leg from above your hip

to your knee. Do not allow your posture to curve forward but keep standing straight up.

4. Hold the stretch for 30 seconds and then relax.
5. Repeat Steps 2–4 four times and then switch to the right quad.

Calf Stretch

We finally have made it down the entire body and you should be feeling loose and great, perhaps even a little tired, since stretching can be hard work. But we're not done yet: We can't forget our calves. They are important in every step we take and look really great when they are in shape.

The calves are actually made up of two muscles: the gastrocnemius, which crosses the knee and ankle, and the soleus, which crosses only the ankle. The ends of the gastroc and soleus tendons fuse in the lower part of the leg as the Achilles tendon. Keeping the calves flexible is not only important for preventing calf tears but for preventing the ever-troublesome Achilles tendinitis or rupture. The Calf Stretch is also very important for women who wear heels all the time. Despite being an orthopaedic surgeon, I am one of these women. (I just can't help it.) We have an added urgency to keep our calves and Achilles tendon flexible because when we wear heels, we walk around with our muscles in a shortened state. Our muscles can actually get so tight and short that we have pain even when walking in flat shoes.

You probably know this stretch already. Make sure that when you do it, you keep the leg straight to stretch your gastrocnemius and bent to stretch your soleus muscle. Both are important.

1. Stand with your feet shoulder-length apart with your hands against a chair or a wall.
2. Take a big step back with each foot, ensuring that they are still shoulder-length apart. Press your heels on the floor and keep your knees straight while leaning into the chair or wall (as shown in Photo 29). You will feel this stretch down the back of your legs (in your gastrocnemius).

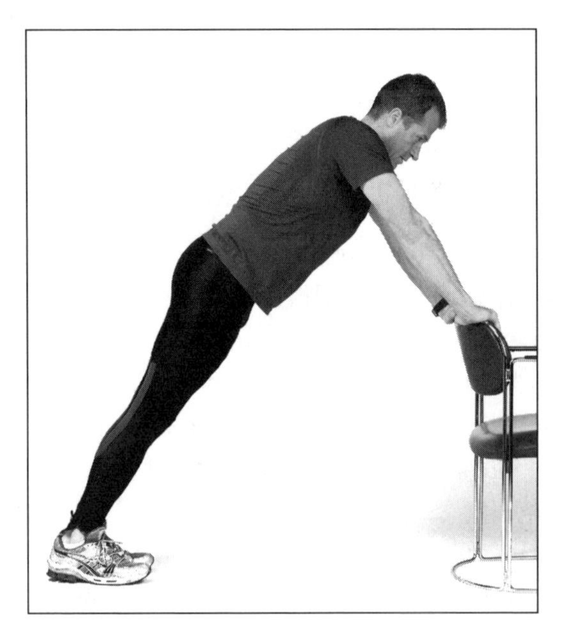

Photo 29

3. Hold the stretch for 30 seconds. Then bend your knees and continue leaning in (as shown in Photo 30). This stretches the deep soleus muscle.
4. Hold the stretch for 30 seconds, then repeat (with both straight and bent knees) four times.

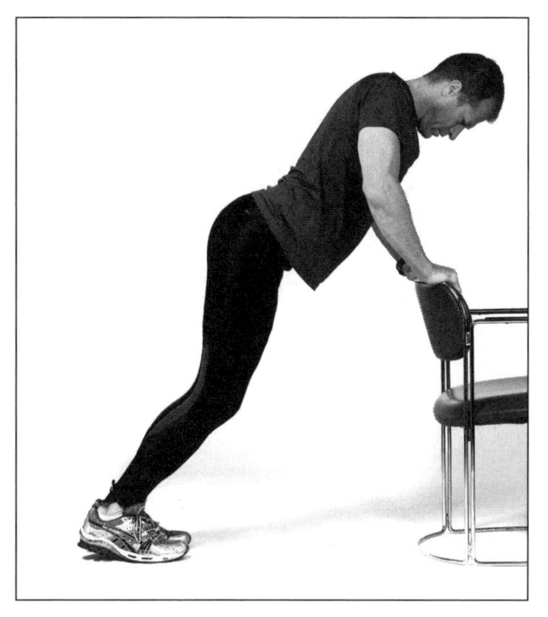

Photo 30

This general stretching program hits all the major muscle groups in the body. As you make stretching a part of your everyday investment in health, you may find that you like doing some of these more than others and may even add things that are not listed here. That is great! It means that you are taking ownership of your body.

HOME**WORK**

The easiest way to adopt my full menu of flexibility boosters is to add a new stretch each day and practice it until it becomes second nature. Start with foam rolling right now. Tomorrow, you should be ready to do both the foam rolling exercises and the Hip Circle (the first exercise in the Dynamic Stretching and Warm-Up sequence). By next week, you'll be ready for Static Stretching. And in six short weeks, you'll be amazed by how much your flexibility has changed!

"So many people spend their health gaining wealth, and then have to spend their wealth to regain their health."

—A. J. Reb Materi

CHAPTER **SEVEN**

7

A—Aerobic Exercise

The fact that your last birthday cake had enough candles to set off the fire alarm does not mean you have to be "old and slow." Neither does 20 years of sedentary living. No age or skill level will impede your body's ability to rise to the opportunity of better health and mobility.

When it comes down to it, mastering fitness after 40 means maximizing performance by working hard enough to sweat. Despite what you may read on newsstands, the secret is not a pill, a fountain, or a magic shot. The process of aging well is neither superficial nor passive. Oh, sure, looking good is as important to me as it is to you, but as your orthopaedic surgeon and mobility doc, I am not really interested in whether you impress friends at your next reunion. Fitness after 40 is not about your dress size. It is about making active decisions *today* and taking control of your health and future at the cellular level *every day*.

Choosing to challenge yourself aerobically is one of those active decisions. It can make the difference in feeling strong and looking good from the inside out. To this end, this chapter gives your aerobic exercise routine a F.A.C.E.-lift by teaching you to maximize your cardiovascular fitness (and therefore health) by being intense in your mobility, using progressive overload and managing your exercise volume to maximize your metabolic returns, and not letting the concept of reversibility ruin your whole game plan.

Make it work, then let it rest. I've found this approach to be very effective for everyone after 40. It borrows aspects of *fartlek* training, which is popular with runners. *Fartlek* is a Swedish word meaning "speed play." This method advocates moving with intensity for a short burst, letting your body recover for a short time, and then repeating the cycle. The beauty of using a speed play approach to aerobic exercise is that no matter your age or fitness level, you can challenge your body to the next level. Even if your personal "intense" is slower than the next guy's, as long as your body recognizes the level of effort you're exerting as intense, you are changing your health from the inside out. Remember, you are in a race with only yourself!

I remember when I was writing the proposal for the first edition of this book. I felt so inspired by what I was writing that I just had to jump up and go for a run. It was one of those rare warm, sunny, beautiful winter days in New York's Central Park. There is a 1.7-mile loop with rolling hills in the south end of the park. As I neared the end of the first loop, I felt great and picked up my pace as I began the second round. It was one of those "out of body" days when I just marveled at how strong I felt. My arms were pumping, my legs were churning, and I was breathing deeply and sweating profusely. I knew that the hard work I had been putting in on the road, in spin class, and carrying a load were clicking in that day! I felt so victorious . . . mastering my 40th year from the inside out.

Now, I'm writing the second edition of *Fitness After 40*. I am running toward my 50th birthday with a bundle of life events (including giving birth) under my belt since the first edition. I am moving toward the next aerobic challenge in my life—running the six races in the World Marathon Majors Series—and using speed play and a more efficient approach to total body fitness. The candles on my birthday cake could burn down my house, but I am not ready to give up intensity, vitality, and feeling strong.

My friends, it is not about your age or your dress size; it is about challenging yourself to live a healthy, vital, active, and joyful today—and every day.

WHAT ABOUT YOU?

Do you think that just because you have celebrated life for a random number of years, you automatically must slow down or stop being active? Remember my study that I discussed in Chapter 2, where I looked at Senior Olympians and found that they maintained a high level of performance? If we are chronically active, biology does not really take over to significantly slow us down until we are in our seventies. The fact is that you are designed to move!

When we were kids, Jabba the Hutt, that blob of meanness from the *Star Wars* film *Return of the Jedi*, had no legs, puny arms, and a gigantic belly that constituted about half of his body. Now *there* was a guy who was not designed to move. Unless you are one of Jabba the Hutt's cousins, movement and activity are in your genes! We are built with strong extremities that respond to activity no matter what our chronologic age.

The key is understanding how you are different now from the way you were when you were 20. Think about being "masterful" as you approach your next 30 or 40 years of activity.

BRING IN THE OXYGEN

In Chapter 6, we talked about staying flexible. The next step in F.A.C.E.-ing your future is getting your heart into the game through aerobic exercise, which means bringing oxygen into the picture. Just as your entire body can put on fat and become weak from disuse, so can your heart. If you don't challenge it, your heart literally becomes surrounded by a flabby envelope of fat and lub-dubs along like a floppy sac.

If you are just beginning to invest in your physical fitness, getting your heart into the game simply means standing up and walking up the stairs instead of taking the escalator or elevator. The pounding you feel in your chest is your heart stepping up to duty. If you already exercise several times a week, the question is whether you are still challenging your heart or whether your usual exercise routine has become too easy.

WHAT IS AEROBIC EXERCISE?

Aerobic means "with oxygen," and aerobic exercise is exercise that involves oxygen. Let's take a step back and understand exactly what happens during aerobic exercise. When you increase your activity level and work your large muscle groups, your muscles require more fuel. Oxygen is the raw material or fuel used to make muscle food, a substance called ATP (adenosine triphosphate, or adenosine 5′-triphosphate). When you exercise, your muscles rapidly pull the oxygen out of your blood. Your brain senses the low oxygen levels and stimulates your body to respond very quickly by making you breathe more rapidly and more deeply. This maximizes the amount of oxygen in your lungs. Oxygen (which makes up 21 percent of the air we breathe) is then passed from your lungs into your blood, where it latches onto hemoglobin molecules. It is then ready for transport to the muscle groups screaming for more fuel. This is where the heart comes in.

Blood that is now filled with oxygen (and thus appears red) moves from your lungs into the left side of your heart. Your heart is a muscle. Like any muscle, the stronger it is, the more efficiently it does its job, and the heart's job is to propel oxygen-rich blood from your lungs to all the tissues of your body.

The left side of your heart fills with blood and then, in a massive contraction, ejects the blood into the arteries that carry the blood to the tissues. (Remember: Arteries move blood *away* from the heart.) When oxygen is delivered to your muscle cells, it is exchanged for cell waste, such as carbon dioxide and lactic acid. The oxygen enters your cells and becomes part of a miraculous and complicated energy-generating system called the Krebs cycle (which, by the way, we all hated memorizing in medical school).

This highly efficient cycle churns out energy in the form of ATP. (If oxygen were crude oil, then ATP is the unleaded gas that goes into our tanks.) Your muscles use ATP for fuel. When your muscles are munching up the fuel faster than your heart can deliver oxygen—or the Krebs cycle can turn it into fuel—the cells switch to a faster, but much less efficient, anaerobic fuel system. This anaerobic (meaning "without oxygen") system is 16 times less efficient than the Krebs cycle and produces the lactic acid that makes your muscles so sore after exercising.

The more fit your body is and the more efficient your heart becomes, the more work it can do with each given amount of oxygen. In other words, if you were a car, the more efficient your heart engine is, the better your miles per gallon or work per unit of oxygen will be.

WHY IS AEROBIC EXERCISE IMPORTANT TO YOU?

If I asked you, you could probably give me 10 or more really good reasons to do aerobic exercise. The problem is not that people don't know that aerobic exercise is the key to aging well. The problem is that only a third of us do 30 minutes of aerobic exercise a day! Where is the disconnect? We all have our reasons. I can assure you that I have heard every conceivable reason (some of which were *very* creative) why my patients don't get off the couch 30 minutes a day and invest in aging well.

We have been talking for a long time about staying fit. Soon, I am going to summarize some important reasons for you to start or increase your aerobic exercise without one more minute of delay. But I feel so strongly about the importance of your not delaying that I would not be offended at all if you put the book down right now and went for a brisk walk, run, row, or bike ride. All of these are fantastic ways to get your heart pumping and your muscles warm. You might also think about removing the pile of stuff cluttering your treadmill or elliptical machine and getting on.

There was a woman in one of my PRIMA Start classes who put on her workout clothes and attended our weekly sessions faithfully. When we meet, we have a 20- to 30-minute lecture about some aspect of fitness and then exercise as a group for the remainder of the time. After five weeks of meeting together, I discovered that when we transitioned from classroom to exercise, this woman would slip away, get in her car, and drive home. She was hoping that she would become inspired enough to exercise by just sitting and listening. In my experience, sitting on the couch or in the classroom and watching and listening does not inspire you to exercise. Real inspiration comes when you get out on the road and sweat. When the program coordinators and I discovered that this woman was not investing in herself, we exercised with her for the next couple of sessions. It was hard for her since she had not challenged herself in years. But at the end of the workouts, she was so proud of her accomplishment. In the same way, I want you to begin exercising while you read this book. Start now and add to your regimen as you read on.

The Reasons for Mobility: What You Already Know

"Getting a move on" in your life is the single most important step (followed closely by quitting smoking) you can do to change your health. Human beings are designed to move. From our stem cells to our musculoskeletal frame to our brain neurons, our bodies crave mobility.

- ***Improve your cardiovascular health***. Multiple studies have proved that physically fit people have a lower death rate than sedentary people. Exercise increases the amount of blood your heart ejects with each beat and the total volume of blood leaving the heart. In turn, this increases the amount and efficiency of oxygen reaching your muscles and organs. Exercise also lowers the heart muscle's demand for oxygen because it uses the oxygen fuel more efficiently.
- ***Lower your risk of diabetes***. Exercise improves the body's response to insulin and lowers the risk of developing diabetes by 30–40 percent. Exercise can also decrease a diabetic's risk of dying of heart disease by 40–50 percent.
- ***Lower your blood pressure***. Many studies have shown that regular exercise lowers your blood pressure, and thus the work your heart has to do. This effect is independent of a person's age or body mass index or the presence of diabetes.
- ***Improve your cholesterol levels***. Exercise increases the level of "good cholesterol" (HDL) in your blood, which acts like Drano to clean out your blood vessels. At the same time, exercise lowers the level of "bad cholesterol" (LDL) and triglycerides (which are dangerous fats) and prevents the bad stuff from sticking to the sides of your blood vessels. Exercise also enhances the beneficial effects of a low-fat diet.
- ***Lower your risk of SeDS***. Although it may sound like a joke, SeDS (Sedentary Death Syndrome) is no laughing matter. The ill effects of more than 33 chronic diseases can be directly decreased by 30 minutes of exercise a day.

The Reasons for Mobility: Amazing Things You May Not Know

If all of these reasons for increasing your mobility were not enough, you might be interested to know that a broad range of new science points to the benefits of exercise on every part of your body.

- ***Improve your brain function***. Exercise makes a type of Miracle-Gro for the brain—really! When you exercise, your brain makes a substance called brain-derived neurotrophic factor (BDNF), which is a type of "brain food." Studies have found that active people are more likely to be better adjusted and perform better on tests of cognitive function. And scientists believe this exercise-induced brain food is the reason.
- ***Lift your mood***. After a stressful day, exercise can calm and improve your mood. According to researchers at the University of Missouri, 30 minutes of moderate to intense aerobic exercise can leave you still feeling on top of the world 90 minutes later. This is because exercise causes the brain to release endorphins, which are natural mood elevators. It's like popping an antidepressant pill but with exercise. People who exercise are 1.5 times less likely to be depressed; they also have higher self-confidence and higher self-esteem than people who do not exercise. This is true for both chronic exercisers and adult-onset exercisers. This effect holds true as long as you are exercising. If you stop exercising, the mood benefits fade with your general fitness. Regular exercise also decreases the cardiac and hormonal responses to mental stress, such as a racing heart, abundant sweating, and feeling on edge.
- ***Improve your erectile functioning***. For some of the same reasons exercise is good for your heart, exercise is great for

sexual function. Physiologically, erection is all about healthy blood flow, and men who exercise have been found to have 41 percent less erectile dysfunction than those who sit on the couch.

- ***Reduce your likelihood of sickness***. Both athlete surveys and randomized studies (done on all sorts of people) have shown that people who do moderate exercise on a near daily basis experience fewer sick days. Exercisers report taking about half the number of sick days as their sedentary peers and having 23 percent fewer upper respiratory tract infections.
- ***Prevent cancer***. Exercise can decrease the risk of breast cancer by up to 60 percent by lowering levels of estradiol and progesterone, two of the ovarian hormones linked to breast cancer. Exercise also can decrease the risk of colorectal cancer by 40 percent and decrease the risk of dying from prostate cancer by 50 percent. If you have or have had cancer, exercise can be of great physical and mental benefit.

THE EXERCISE-CANCER CONNECTION

Exercise offers many physical and mental benefits that deter cancer, especially breast and prostate cancer. If you have or have had breast cancer, research suggests that a few hours of walking or other exercise each week may help you live longer. In the study, done at Harvard University of nearly 3,000 women, those who exercised the equivalent of walking about one hour a week at a pace of two to three miles per hour had a lower risk of dying from breast cancer than women who got less than an hour's worth of physical activity each week. Women who did a little more than that—the equivalent of walking about three to five hours per week at the same pace—had the lowest risk of dying. Women who got more exercise than that also had a lower risk of dying, but not as low as women in the middle group.[1] In short, doing three to five hours of physical activity is better than straining to do more.

This finding could give you another way to boost your odds of beating breast cancer. "Women with breast cancer have little to lose and much to gain from exercise," said the study's lead author, Michelle Holmes, of Harvard Medical School and Brigham and Women's Hospital in Boston. "We already know that [breast cancer patients who exercise] have better mood, better body image, and better self-esteem. We know it [exercise] fights other diseases that women with breast cancer can also get, like heart disease and diabetes. And it may also help these women avoid dying from breast cancer."[2]

The same benefits from exercise hold true for men with prostate cancer. Decreased physical activity, which may be the result of the cancer itself or the treatment for it, can lead to tiredness and lack of energy. Results of the Health Professionals Follow-Up Study of 47,000 men over a 14-year period, published in the *Archives of Internal Medicine* in 2005, showed that men over age 65 who engaged in at least three hours of vigorous physical activity (such as running, biking, or swimming) per week had a nearly 70 percent lower risk of being diagnosed with advanced prostate cancer or dying from the disease.[3] Researchers say more study is needed to understand how exercise affects prostate cancer risk in men of all ages, but these findings show that vigorous exercise may slow the progression of prostate cancer in older men.

In another finding, by researchers at UCLA's Jonsson Comprehensive Cancer Center and Department of Physiological Science, a low-fat, high-fiber diet and regular exercise reportedly slowed prostate cancer cell growth by up to 30 percent. Study participants walked at 70–85 percent of their maximum heart rate four to five times per week for 30 to 60 minutes, and once or twice a week at a slower pace for 40 to 60 minutes. "This is the first study to directly measure the effects of diet and exercise on inhibiting prostate cancer cell growth," said William Aronson, senior author of the study. "We used a new method, developed by our research team, to evaluate how effectively these lifestyle changes might help slow the growth of prostate cancer cells, and we are extremely encouraged by the results."[4]

HOW DO I START?

Getting started should be as easy as putting on a pair of shoes and going out for a walk around the block. To optimize your safety, especially if you are an AOE (or have an exercise history that begins "Once upon a time . . ."), you should take these steps to ensure your safety.

Check In with Your Doctor

If you are just beginning to exercise, read the seven questions listed below. This is a simple checklist, designed by the Canadian Society for Exercise Physiology, to determine whether or not you need to check with your doctor to receive medical clearance to exercise. When in doubt, however, always see your doctor.

1. Has your doctor ever said that you have a heart condition and that you should do only physical activity recommended by a doctor?
2. Do you feel pain in your chest when you do physical exercise?

3. In the past month, have you had chest pain when you were not doing exercise?
4. Do you lose your balance because of dizziness, or do you ever lose consciousness?
5. Do you have a bone or joint problem that could be made worse by a change in your physical activity?
6. Is your doctor currently prescribing drugs for you for blood pressure or a heart condition?
7. Do you know of any other reason why you should not do physical activity?

If you answered *no* to all seven questions, you can be reasonably sure that you can start becoming more physically active if you start slowly and build up gradually. You could also participate in a community fitness appraisal to determine your basic fitness level. Many community health centers, YMCAs, or gyms bring in medical personnel to perform these health overviews. Be aware that if you answered *no* to all of the questions because you have not been to the doctor in years, then now is the time to get checked out.

If you answered *yes* to one or more of the above questions, you should talk to your doctor by phone or in person before starting to increase your activity. You may still be able to do any activity you want by starting slowly and increasing gradually. However, your doctor will have the opportunity to discuss the activities you'd like to participate in. In addition, the American Heart Association recommends that anyone with known heart disease see his doctor prior to beginning an exercise program.

When you visit your doctor, she will interview you and review the cardiovascular risk factors listed in the section on these factors. An electrocardiogram (EKG) may be done to look at your heart function. If you have a moderate- to high-risk profile for heart disease, have known cardiovascular disease, or are older than 65 even with no risk factors, your doctor may also want to perform an exercise stress test.

CARDIOVASCULAR RISK FACTORS

Moderate cardiac risk is defined as men 40 to 45 years old or women 50 to 55 years old with one or more of the following:

- Total cholesterol of more than 200 mg/dL
- LDL (low-density lipoprotein—the "bad cholesterol") of more than 130 mg/dL
- HDL (high-density lipoprotein—the "good cholesterol") of less than 40 mg/dL
- High blood pressure of more than 140/90 mm Hg
- Current or recent cigarette smoking
- Diabetes or fasting blood sugar of less than 126 mg/dL
- A history of sudden cardiac death in a member of your immediate family who was less than 60 years old

Determine What "Intense" Means to You

How do we know when we are exercising enough (aerobically with oxygen) and not too much (anaerobically without oxygen)? For an effective workout, you need to exercise within your target heart rate and stay there for 20 minutes or more. Raising your heart rate and keeping it up burns fat and increases your cardiovascular fitness. In other words, you build a lean, efficient cardio engine.

To pinpoint the level of intensity that is right for you, many experts recommend determining your maximum heart rate (or MaxHR) and then working out at 85 percent of this number. When you reach this level of intensity during a workout, you are not able to have a conversation. More importantly, 85 percent of your MaxHR is the level at which our efficient aerobic metabolism switches to the less efficient, but more rapid, anaerobic metabolism (or "lactate threshold"). Some researchers hold that there is no true MaxHR and that our capacity for cardiovascular fitness is determined by fitness level, age, heart size, ambient (surrounding) temperature, and even current hydration status. Nevertheless, MaxHR remains an estimate for determining how intensely you should be working out.

You can calculate your target heart rate by following these three steps:

1. Determine your MaxHR. (More about this below.)
2. Multiply your MaxHR by 0.85. This is your maximum target rate.
3. Multiply your MaxHR by 0.50. This is your minimum target rate.

The most common way to calculate MaxHR is simply to subtract your age from 220. However, this is an inaccurate method; it can be up to 40bpm (beats per minute) off after age 30. A more accurate method was published by the K. G. Jebsen Center for Exercise in Medicine at the Norwegian University of Science and Technology after studying more than 3,000 people ages 19 to 89. They determined that MaxHR is more accurately determined by the following formula: 211 – (.64 x Age); in other words, 211 minus 64 percent of a person's age. This formula carries a standard deviation of +/– 10bpm.

If you are 50 years old, your MaxHR is 211 – (.64 x 50), or 179bpm. Multiplying 179 by 0.85 gives you a maximum target rate of 152bpm. Multiplying 179 by 0.50 gives you a minimum target rate of 89bpm. Thus, your target heart range is between 89 and 152bpm.

You can use your target heart rate to help achieve your goals. Working out at 60–70 percent of your MaxHR is best for weight management and a fit appearance; 70–80 percent puts you in the heart-healthy aerobic zone; and 80–100 percent gives you the competitive edge for peak performance.

During your workouts, periodically check your heart rate. If you have a heart rate monitor (a device worn on your chest and wrist that can detect and track your heart rate while you are active), you can set the alarm limits around your target heart range.

If you do not have a monitor, you can get a rough estimate of your heart rate by counting your pulse for six seconds and adding a zero. You can check your pulse by placing your index and middle fingers lightly on your radial pulse. This is the pulse on the thumb side of your wrist. Press lightly, because pressing too heavily cuts off the flow of blood through the vessel, and you will be unable to count. You can also place your fingers lightly on either side of your windpipe (the hard tube in the very center of your throat) to feel your carotid pulse. Do not press too hard or massage this area, since this can affect your heart rate. Practice taking your pulse before you start to exercise so you know what you are feeling for before you exercise. If your heart rate is too slow, pick up your pace; if it is too high, then slow down a bit.

If you continually exercise above your target range, your heart may not be able to keep up with your oxygen demand, and you will switch from the efficient aerobic form of exercise to the inefficient anaerobic form. The anaerobic form produces lactic acid as a by-product and makes you feel sore.

As you get into shape, your target heart rate will not change. However, the work that you have to do to get your heart into that range will change. The better shape you are in, the more efficient your heart is and the lower your resting heart rate will become. You will have to put forth more effort to raise your heart rate. For instance, when you first step away from the couch, it may take only a moderately paced walk to get your heart into the 60–70 percent of MaxHR zone. As you become more fit, however, you may need to walk briskly or even jog to get your heart rate up. Your heart has become more efficient and does more work with each stroke.

Here is an example of how to use workout time and target heart rate together. Let's say you are running on a track for 30 minutes. When you begin to exercise, you may be able to run only four laps and keep your heart in the target range. As you become more fit, however, you may be able increase your speed and cover five laps or eventually six laps in the same time period without working outside your target heart range. By now, you will be feeling a noticeable change in your daily stamina, state of mind, and energy level. As you get in better shape, you can increase the intensity or the duration of your workout. You will find that as you increase the duration of your aerobic activity, your heart rate may go up toward the end. This is the effect of fatigue. When your heart rate remains in the target zone until the end of your workout, then it is time to increase the amount of workout time or intensity again.

For those of you already working out, you can increase your performance by increasing the intensity of your workout from 60–70 percent to 70–80 percent of your MaxHR. (You can calculate this as explained above.) Once you are able to move through your workout comfortably at this intensity, you can continue improving by adding time or distance. For instance, you can increase your aerobic period from 30 to 45 minutes or increase the intensity of your 30-minute workout to 70–80 percent of your MaxHR. If long-distance running (a marathon or a half marathon) is your goal, you should build your endurance base in the 60–70 percent MaxHR zone. This means that while your shorter midweek runs can be 70–80 percent intense, those long weekend runs should slow down to 60–70 percent intense.

A fun way to improve your fitness is to do *fartlek* runs. As mentioned earlier, *fartlek* is a Swedish word that means "speed play." This method of increasing your workout intensity alternates running at an easy pace with running at your MaxHR. *Fartleks* allow you to work out without getting tired because as soon as you reach the upper limit of your MaxHR, you immediately slow down to walk or jog until your heart rate recovers. An example of a *fartlek* would be starting with a one-mile jog at 60–70 percent effort. When you reach this point, you pick up your speed and run faster or even sprint until your heart reaches 85 percent of your MaxHR, and then you immediately slow down again until your heart rate returns to 60–70 percent. You then speed up again. You keep alternating slow/fast for a set period of time (20 or 30 minutes, for example) and increase the intensity of the workout by increasing the duration. This is a great way to work from walking to running.

The speed play method actually works well no matter which type of aerobic exercise you choose each day. I recommend warming up for five to 10 minutes with the Dynamic Stretching and Warm-Up (discussed in Chapter 6). For the first speed play interval, move at a pace that exerts 60–70 percent effort for three minutes, then increase your intensity to 85 percent for two minutes. Immediately back off to your recovery pace (60–70 percent effort) for three minutes, followed by a two-minute intense (85 percent effort) period. Continue these five-minute speed plays for 20 to 30 minutes. You can also perform speed play aerobic workouts using landmarks or laps instead of clocking your time.

To begin your own exercise program, choose the aerobic activity you are going to start doing, such as walking, hiking, running, jogging, aerobic dance, rope skipping, stairs, skating, cycling, skiing, aerobics classes, rowing, swimming, or endurance sports. Keep track of what your heart is doing. I find that the easiest way to track what my heart is doing and be precise about my workouts is to wear a heart rate monitor.

Keep It Simple

When you are getting started, it is important to keep it simple. Do not make an elaborate plan with multilevel goals. Go for a walk, run, swim, or row—anything that is logistically practical for you. Remember that just making the decision to exercise does not erase years of sedentary buildup, so don't try to make it up all at once. Many people start with walking first, since you can just open the front door and start. And let's face it, there is no new skill to learn.

In addition to making the activity simple, you also need to be very specific when you are planning your upcoming launch into activity. Know the activity, the day, and the time in which you will participate in it, as well as what you hope to accomplish before you begin. Write it down in your calendar or set an alarm on your phone.

Being strategic in your planning is very important. You strategically plan every day in business, your finances, and your social activities. Why not apply the same discipline that works in other parts of your life to caring for your body? A daily strategic plan might read: *Saturday at 3:30 P.M.: Walk in North Park for 35 minutes with my heart rate at 65 percent MaxHR*. Make a plan for each day of the week, even if the plan for Sunday says: *Rest and restore all day*.

In Chapter 10, you will find suggestions on how to make a six-week plan. Each of the weeks should have a strategic plan where you reward yourself. Place your workout plan prominently in your life, posting it on your refrigerator, bathroom mirror, computer calendar, and so on.

Warm Up

You must *always* warm up before taking off on your exercise adventure. This can take the form of an easy walk or a slow jog before a run, or a few slow pool laps before you turn up the speed. Dynamic Stretching and Warm-Ups—warm-ups where you are moving and stretching instead of just standing in one place—are fun and get the heart pumping and the muscles filled with blood. The foam rolling and dynamic stretching exercises in Chapter 6 detail my approach to warming up for a great aerobic workout. Make sure to start with these to maximize your aerobic workout. A great way to get the most out of your Dynamic Stretching and Warm-Up is to jog/walk for 20–30 yards between each exercise set.

Take 10,000 Steps

Are you just stepping away from the couch after years of sedentary living? One easy way to increase the overall activity in your life is to use the 10,000-step method. In this method, which originated in Japan, you monitor the activity you do during a day, making you conscious of the number of steps you take. Then you try to increase your activity and number of steps. To do this you need a pedometer, which you can buy in most sporting goods stores; some are even given away at workplaces.

Wear the pedometer when you go out the door in the morning, and keep it on as you do your usual activities. When you go to bed at night, take it off and record the number of steps you took. Do this for a week. I think you will be surprised to learn how much or how little you actually travel in one day using your own two feet.

A sedentary person usually covers only 1,000 to 3,000 steps per day traveling from place to place—from and to his house, car, workplace, and any businesses patronized for errands. This is not enough to cause meaningful changes in your fitness level. If you find that your baseline falls in this range, you can increase your activity each day by increasing the number of steps you take.

But what is the big deal with taking a lot of steps, you ask? Many of us spend our workday at a sedentary job. Research has shown that people who work in a seated position for most of the day have a higher risk of dying from cardiac disease than people in the same industry who have more active jobs: Bus drivers are more at risk than train conductors, for example, and postal clerks are more at risk than postal delivery people. In addition, executives who rest all weekend are more at risk than executives who participate in vigorous exercise on weekends. The findings applied whether or not the people had other risk factors—high blood pressure, smoking, obesity, or family history. What this means is that even if you have one of the four other major causes of cardiac disease, activity can still decrease your risk!

To become more fit and control chronic disease, we need to take 10,000 steps a day. If the average person has a stride length of 2.5 feet, this means that it takes about 2,000 steps to cover a mile; 10,000 steps a day would then be about five miles of activity. This can include your 30 minutes of aerobic activity and usually must in order to get that many steps in.

I found this was true for me. When I lived in New York and didn't have a car, I would walk to work, the store, the gym, restaurants . . . everywhere I needed to go. But I found that unless I actually went for a run, I did not accumulate 10,000 steps. I lived a mile from Central Park and would walk there, run three miles, and walk back and still have only about 6,500 steps on my pedometer. That meant I needed my usual daily walking plus a workout to get enough activity.

If you are going to use a pedometer and count your steps, don't get discouraged. Ten thousand steps is a nice round number to aim for, but if your goal is only to prevent weight gain, you may not need to log that many steps. You can build up gradually and be more active on some days than on others. What is most important is that you are off the couch!

Use Time (Not Distance) When You Begin

When you begin your workout, you may want to use time as the measure of your work initially instead of distance. For instance, if you are going to start your workout by walking, begin at a comfortable pace for 10 minutes to warm up. Then stop and do the leg stretching exercises you learned in Chapter 6. Alternatively, you can do the Dynamic Stretching and Warm-Up. When you are warmed up, begin exercising again at a pace that elevates your heart rate to within your target range. This means that, unless you have a heart rate monitor, you may have to stop momentarily to take your pulse, but that's okay. If you are working hard enough, you should recognize your aerobic system kicking in. Your breathing will get quicker and deeper and you may feel your heart beating faster in your chest. Continue exercising for at least 20 minutes. It's okay if you need to slow down or even stop to rest initially.

Over the next several weeks, build up to a continuous 20 minutes of exercise. When you are able to do this, increase your workout by two to five minutes each week until you are able to do 30 continuous minutes within your target heart rate zone. I encourage you to use the principles discussed in this chapter for increasing your activity level and volume.

Think about how you would like to use your workout time, and make a plan that will work for you. This way, the plan belongs to you and you are more likely to adhere to it. If, however, you would like to use a simple plan that works with my patients, you can follow along in Chapter 10.

Move Forward with Progressive Overload

Our bodies are amazingly adaptable machines! To maximize any performance (from stepping off the couch to winning your race), you must carefully and consistently increase the intensity of your movement—in other words, progressively overload your body—whether you are doing aerobic exercise or carrying a load.

Many times people who come to my office proudly tell me that for years they have been walking two miles every day with their friends. I think this is great and definitely better than living a totally sedentary life! Any way we get mobility into our lives, from fidgeting to walking, improves our health.

The fact is, however, if you have been walking the same route with the same friends at the same pace for years, it is not the best thing you can be doing for your health. Our bodies require a certain amount of stress (sweat, increased heart rate, intensity) to trigger the adaptive mechanisms—in our muscles, tendons, bones, brains, and even our genes—that maximize our health.

Simply put, you must work harder every day to see the health benefits of your efforts. This means increasing the volume, intensity, and frequency of your workout over time. This progressive overload can take the form of perfecting your exercise form, increasing the frequency of your normal workouts, increasing the volume of one component at a time, doing the same workout faster, and so forth. This good stress will trigger the adaptive mechanisms in your body to increase the size, density, strength, and neuromuscular control of your muscles, bones, and organs—as well as increase the blood supply to all.

There is no one-size-fits-all way to progressively overload your system, but the speed play intervals (discussed previously in this chapter) and the 20 Minutes to Burn circuits (detailed in Chapter 10) are a great way to progressively overload your body and trigger maximum performance while minimizing injury.

Use It (or You Really Will Lose It!)

"Use it or lose it" is not just a clever cliché but a research-proven principle of health. If you don't trigger your body's adaptive mechanisms for maximizing health through mobility, your body will begin to decondition in as few as two days. *Ouch!*

The physical and mental gains we achieve from mobility and investing every day in our fitness after 40 will inevitably have peaks and valleys, starts and stops, but even after as few as two days without the good stress of exercise, we begin to switch off the genes that guide our cells and bodies toward maximum life and switch on the genes that lead to dormancy and minimized health. Basically, a sedentary lifestyle tells our bodies that we are living at a sustenance level and that even some of our most vital organs, such as muscle and bone, are dispensable. Imagine: If we start at peak shape and then, for whatever reason, take a two-month hiatus, we lose 10 percent of our muscle mass and up to 40 percent of our endurance. All that hard work vanished. Even a weekend warrior turns into a weak-end warrior.

Throughout *Fitness After 40*, I advocate "making it work and letting it rest." This means you should work one body part or body system intensely one day and then either rest to recover or work a different body part the next day. I know all this talk of intense attention to F.A.C.E.-ing your future can be daunting, but I believe that you are worth the daily investment in your health. You are important!

WHAT 15 MINUTES CAN DO FOR YOU

Before you start to say "I just don't have time," look around. I know you can find 15 minutes once, twice, or three times a day. Look at what you can accomplish in 15 minutes:

Activity	Calories Burned
Stair climbing	150
Running	150
Jumping rope	150
Shoveling snow	120
Playing football	120
Playing tennis	100
Walking	75
Bicycling	75
Swimming	75
Washing floors	70
Dancing	70
Doing light housework	60 to 70
Working at your desk	30
Sleeping	18
Watching TV	18

WHY ARE YOU EXERCISING?

You need to answer an important question about your activity: Why are you exercising? What is the point of your activity? Is it to get better at the activity and get in shape, or just to continue to do what comes easily to you? If the point is to improve, then challenge yourself and take it up to the next level.

I was having a discussion with *New York Times* journalist Gina Kolata about why men seem more likely to challenge themselves to the next level of fitness than women (a topic for another time). As we were talking, she mentioned an insightful comment her 17-year-old son had made to her: "Mom, why are you running, anyway?" He did not mean that she should list the 30 good reasons to get and stay in shape. Instead, he wanted to know why, after all this time, she was still jogging along at a pace that now felt like a walk in the park.

I can identify with this question, too. For years, I ran at the same pace because it was easy. My goal was to get through a long run without really breathing hard. Not until I worked out more smartly and intensely did I drop my time per mile. For me, it was a mind-blowing and very proud moment when I crossed the UAE Healthy Kidney 10K run (held in New York City each year) at an average pace of 7:44 per mile (even with a pit stop). That intensity is not going to win me any Olympic medals, but I'm in a race with myself, and that was better than any race I had run since high school. I've come to a place in my workout life where if I'm not challenging myself, I don't see the point at all.

Where are you? Why are you working out?

HOME**WORK**

Take the following actions for your health *right now*:

- Make a doctor's appointment to get cleared to go. Give your physician a copy of this book so she knows your plan.
- Determine your resting and maximum heart rate.
- Jump-start your health with some speed play (*fartlek*). Don't wait. Try it *now!*

NOTES

1. Holmes, Michelle D., Wendy Y. Chen, Diane Feskanich, Candyce H. Kroenke, and Graham A. Colditz, "Physical Activity and Survival After Breast Cancer Diagnosis," *JAMA* 293(20): 2479–2486 (2005).

2. American Cancer Society, "Exercise Can Improve Breast Cancer Survival," www.aahf.info/sec_news/section/bc_survival_081105.htm.

3. Giovannucci, Edward L., Yan Liu, Michael F. Leitzmann, Meir J. Stampfer, and Walter C. Willett, "A Prospective Study of Physical Activity and Incident and Fatal Prostate Cancer," *Archives of Internal Medicine* 165(9): 1005–1010 (2005).

4. UniSci, "Diet, Exercise Slow Prostate Cancer as Much as 30 Percent," www.unisci.com/stories/20013/0911013.htm.

"I'm just totally into being strong. There's something about wanting to get a jar or whatever out of a high cupboard, or moving a sofa over because my dog's bone rolled under it, and not having to call anyone for help. There's comfort in that."

—Maggie Q, film and television actress

CHAPTER **EIGHT** 8

C—Carry a Load

What is carrying a load? It simply means resistance training, but preferably not on stationary weight machines. Pushing and pulling weight around is vital for fitness after 40. If aging progresses unchecked, we lose 10 percent of our muscle mass between the ages of 25 and 50, and 45 percent more between the ages of 50 and 80. This loss of lean muscle mass (sarcopenia) leaves us vulnerable to falls, poor bone health, and an inability to do the things we want to do physically each day. The great news is that when it comes to lean muscle mass, if we use it, we can prevent its loss—and stay strong!

To stave off muscle decline, you *must* carry a load. This has other benefits, too. Not only does it make you look great but it keeps your bones strong, lowers your blood pressure, and may reduce the risk of stroke. In addition, muscle burns more calories during activities of daily living than fat. If you build up your muscles so that a great percentage of your body is muscle rather than fat, you will use more calories by simply living than you did when you had less muscle and more fat. In addition, maintaining and building muscle is good for your metabolism, makes you strong, prevents falling, curtails injury, and lifts your mood. Because loss of muscle increases markedly after age 50, lifting weights after 50 is critical.

I specifically do not call this activity "weight lifting" because I am not talking about going to a gym, sitting on a machine, and lifting a stack of weights off the rack. To build functional strength for both sports and everyday life, we need to strengthen our muscles in the way we actually use them. This means optimal resistance training—moving weight through a range of motions with gravity and ground reactive forces pushing back on us just like in real life. In addition, in life we never use just one muscle to lift an object or move our bodies. We need total body strength.

Let me give you an example: Many of us grew up in an era when "strengthening our quadriceps" meant sitting on a leg press machine and pushing a sled of weight up a slope away from our bodies. While this can make your quads stronger, when was the last time in real life you used your leg muscles to push a load of weight up a slope while sitting on your butt? The fact is that you use your quads in coordination with your core, butt, hamstrings, and so forth to squat down and pick up an object or even your kids or grandkids.

We should train our muscles to function in the way we use them, in coordination with the rest of the muscles in our body. Instead of sitting on a leg press machine, you should do Short Arc Wall Squats, Prisoner Squats, or even a variety of lunges to build total body strength. (Short Arc Wall Squats and Prisoners Squats are described later in this chapter.)

I am often shocked when I see the X-rays of one of my patient's legs. X-rays are for looking at bones, but they show shadows of the soft tissues around the bones. Sometimes there is only a thin layer of muscle surrounding the bone and a thick layer of fat under the skin. This can be the case for both heavy people and thin people if they are not strong. We need strong, thick muscles to do everything from getting out of a chair to climbing a flight of stairs, from preventing falls to jogging around the block. Just because a person looks in the mirror and sees a thick thigh does not mean that he has enough muscle to support his bones and joints. On the other hand, thin does not mean fit. Thin can mean that there is not enough muscle.

With muscle, you truly lose it if you don't use it. Have you ever had your arm or leg in a cast? Do you remember how tight the cast was against your skin when the doctor put it on? Perhaps it even felt confining and uncomfortable. Within a week or so, however, the cast became looser, and you could see clear space between it and your skin. This was the result of disuse atrophy of the muscle. Essentially, this is what happens to your entire body if you don't actively use your muscles.

Once your muscle is lost, do you weigh less? No. The five pounds of muscle we lose is typically replaced with five pounds of fat. This fat makes us bigger all around because a pound of fat takes up 18 percent more room on our frame than a pound of muscle.

There are countless articles in the medical and exercise physiology literature that document the fact that muscle disuse atrophy is reversible in both mature athletes and aging couch potatoes. In as few as eight to 12 weeks, resistance training can produce marked improvements in strength and endurance.

One classic study from 1993 looked at two groups of masters athletes. One group ran 30 minutes three times per week, while the other group ran 15 minutes three times per week and carried a load with all their major muscle groups for the remaining 15 minutes. At the end of four months, bone density and lean muscle mass increased significantly in the group that did resistance work as well as running, while bone density and lean muscle mass did not increase in the group that only went running.

With a low-repetition/high-weight regimen, both masters athletes and active agers can show similar or greater strength gains compared with younger people. A two- to three-fold increase in muscle strength can be accomplished in a relatively short period of time (12 weeks) with moderately intense workouts. In addition, heavy resistance training improves the amount of protein your body retains no matter how much you eat. Even people eating lower-protein diets can build muscle when they lift weights because they retain more of what they eat.

Many studies document much greater muscle mass, architecture, and functional strength in strength-trained masters athletes than in their sedentary peers. However, not only the *quantity* of the muscle improves; the *quality* improves as well. These benefits are dependent on the intensity of the exercise performed. This means that lifting heavier weights is better than lifting lighter weights.

Strength training has other benefits as well. For instance, as we age it is an important part of weight management. It is also associated with increased energy requirements during rest, which simply means that you use more energy just to live if you have more muscle. How many more calories? Research in the Netherlands documented a 9 percent greater calorie burn with resistance training. Even without diet changes, this translates into lost pounds. A big bonus of strength training is also more effective insulin sensitivity for people with diabetes. The more muscle you have, the better your body responds to the insulin you take or make by lowering your blood sugar. A true weekly weight program can decrease insulin levels by 25 percent after a high-carbohydrate meal. Finally, carrying a load not only strengthens bone and increases muscle mass and strength, but the combination of these factors decreases the incidence of falls and thus osteoporotic fractures (fractures that occur because of weak bone).

Lifting weights may evoke images of big, sweaty guys hoisting iron plates onto sagging metal crossbars and grunting out the effort as they push the weight around. Carrying a load does not, however, have to be a burden, and you do not have to do endless repetitions of heavy weights to receive a benefit. In fact, it is not necessary to haul steel around at all. One of the best "loads" to carry is your own body weight.

HOW TO CARRY A LOAD

When carrying a load, start by working the large muscle groups, and then progress to the smaller ones. You can begin with your legs or arms. With the legs, begin with your buttocks or quadriceps before moving down the leg to the smaller calf muscles. With the arms, begin with the pectoralis (chest), biceps, triceps, and so forth, before moving to the smaller rotator cuff muscles in the upper arm. This way, you get the most demanding work out of the way when you are not so tired. How fast you move through the lift is also important. Lifting should be slow and controlled, never jerking.

There are a lot of different ways to carry a load. It is not necessary to have access to a weight machine. Free weights—such as dumbbells, exercise bands, and your own body—are all excellent weights to carry. (More on exercise bands—also called resistance bands—which look like heavy-duty rubber bands, in a few paragraphs.) Some strength coaches actually prefer free weights and exercise bands over stationary machines because they require you to engage the pathways between your brain and muscles to control and balance the weights. Don't forget: In this age of high-tech gym equipment, it can be highly effective just to lift your own upper body weight with push-ups and chin-ups and your lower body weight with Short Arc Wall Squats (described later in this chapter).

Research has shown that you can receive 60 percent of the total benefit from resistance training by doing one set of eight to 10 repetitions per muscle group two to three times per week. And you can receive more than 80 percent of the benefit by doing two sets. Each repetition should be between 60 and 85 percent of the maximum weight you are able to lift one time, or your "one-rep max."

To find your one-rep max, simply keep increasing the weight until you can do only one repetition of the load. Make sure you are not jerking the weight, since you could hurt yourself. If you are using exercise bands, progress up in thickness until you are using the one that is hardest for you to stretch. (Exercise bands come in different colors to indicate different levels of resistance. Generally, they progress from yellow, which is the lightest, to red, green, blue, gray, and black, which is the heaviest. In addition, some exercise bands—called continuous bands—come as a loop, while others are just straight and must be tied into a loop for certain exercises.)

Once you determine your maximum weight for a muscle group, calculate what 70–80 percent of that is. This is your workout weight. For instance, I can curl 20 pounds with my left (nondominant) bicep one time, and 80 percent of that is 16 pounds. Therefore, I work out with a 15-pound dumbbell (there is no 16-pound dumbbell), and I do one set of 10 repetitions. Remember that with one set, you get 60 percent of the benefit, and with two sets, you get more than 80 percent. I have settled on one set because of time constraints; one set is sufficient to keep my arms strong and fit.

Lifting more than 85 percent of your maximum can increase your risk of injury, while lifting less than 60 percent is not effective. This means that the total number of reps can be low, but the weight should be intense. Each repetition should be taken through a full range of motion in a slow, controlled move. You should take twice as long to lower the weight as you do to lift it. For instance, you can do Biceps Curls (described later in this chapter) with either a free weight or tubing. (Resistance tubes are like large rubber bands that you pull. Depending on their size, they offer different degrees of resistance and therefore the amount of work your muscles do. Like exercise bands, they come in a variety of colors, with each representing a different resistance strength. Different brands come in a rainbow variety of colors that do not remain consistent across all brands. You will need to test out the specific set you choose. You should start with a color that you have to work to pull but that is not so resistant that it hurts or that you cannot complete a set of 10.) When you do Biceps Curls, if you lift the weight by bending your elbow for two seconds, then you should take four seconds to extend your elbow and lower the weight. Do not jerk the weight up; this is a good way to tear your musculotendonous junction (the connection between your muscles and your tendons).

When you have been using one weight level for a while, lifting may become easy. This is called adaptation. To continue getting stronger, you must increase the weight you are lifting. It is time to increase the weight when you can easily lift your current weight 12 times. You can then progress your weight by 5 percent and decrease your number of repetitions to eight.

Remember that when you are standing in front of the mirror watching your muscles flex and bulge, you will not see them getting bigger. During active weight lifting, you are actually creating tiny microtears in the muscle substance. During your rest periods every other day between workouts, your muscles repair and rebuild to increase in size and strength. This is one of the reasons why I always say "make it work and then let it rest."

In this second edition of *Fitness After 40*, I have added 24 new exercises to this chapter as well as included an entirely new chapter, Chapter 10, that features total body circuits for you to carry a load with your body weight or free weights. The 20 Minutes to Burn workouts in Chapter 10 integrate your total body, gravity, and ground reactive forces to build functional strength in the way you actually use your muscles in everyday life.

MUSCLE GROUPS TO COVER IN YOUR WEIGHT TRAINING

To optimize your strength, focus not only on the cosmetic muscles that you can see in the mirror in the gym but—most importantly—on your small supporting muscles.

Your Upper Extremities

- *Latissimi dorsi*. The two big muscles that form a V across your back.
- *Rotator cuff*. A group of four small muscles (supraspinatus, infraspinatus, subscapularis, and teres minor) that provide shoulder stability by keeping your arm bone (the humerus) centered in the socket. Your rotator cuff is the key to shoulder health.
- *Biceps*. The "guns" in the front of your upper arm.

Triceps. The gun balancers in the back of your upper arm.

Deltoid muscles. Your shoulder caps.

Wrist extensors. Muscles in the back of your lower arm.

Wrist flexors. Muscles in the front of your lower arm.

Your Core

- *Rectus abdominis*. The center line of muscles down your front, commonly referred to as a "six pack."
- *Oblique abdominals*. Two muscle sheets wrapping around your waist, from your back to your front. They are the keys to core stability and back health and are responsible for trunk rotation.
- *Transverse abdominis*. The muscles that allow compression of your abdomen.
- *Erector spinae*. The muscles that support your spine and stabilize trunk extension.
- *Multifidus*. The small posterior muscles that control your spine stability.

Your Lower Extremities

- *Buttocks (the three gluteus muscles)*. The muscles that provide pelvic stability as well as acceleration and deceleration of motion.
- *Hip flexors*. The muscles (iliopsoas) that flex your hip up.
- *Quadriceps*. Four large muscles in the front of your thighs that are the key to healthy knees.
- *Hamstrings*. Muscles in the back of your thighs that flex your knees.
- *Anterior tibialis*. A muscle in the front of your shin responsible for ankle flexion.
- *Gastrocnemius*. One of the two muscle layers in your calves.

INTRODUCING FITNESS TO GO

The beauty of the Fitness to Go concept (and the 40 resistance exercises that follow) is that the exercises are 100 percent portable. You don't need special machines to do them, and you can take them with you when you travel for business or pleasure. You can hang exercise bands from your office door and get in a few sets between clients, or you can keep the bands around the house and work in a set whenever you have a free minute. You can even stick the bands in your purse and work out on the go!

Many of the Fitness to Go exercises on the pages that follow are incorporated into the 20 Minutes to Burn exercise bricks. These bricks are key components of the Six-Week Jump Start to Mobility Plan in Chapter 10.

You may have performed many of the weight-lifting maneuvers found on the following pages at some point in your life, so they may be familiar to you. In addition, Fitness to Go offers one final but very important bonus: It covers the key focus areas for preventing and minimizing injury (as detailed in the section "Preventing and Minimizing Key Injuries After 40"). Doing these exercises will preemptively strengthen the muscle groups most susceptible to injury and prepare you for sports battle.

PREVENTING AND MINIMIZING KEY INJURIES AFTER 40

After taking care of athletes and active people for the last 29 years, I know that injury often accompanies activity. This is either because of the "Terrible Toos" (too much, too soon, too often, and with too little rest), because our technique and exercise form leaves us open to injury, or simply because of muscle imbalances and weakness we need to address. The four most common areas of complaint that weekend warriors and active agers bring to my office are as follows:

1. Leg and ankle tendinitis 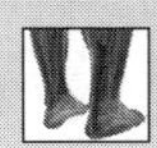
2. Knee pain 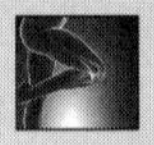
3. Lower back pain 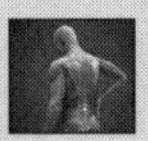
4. Shoulder pain 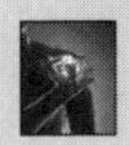

Many of the Fitness to Go exercises featured on the pages that follow are specifically designed to prevent problems in these four key areas. Simply look for the icon that corresponds to the area that you are concerned about and design your individualized workout plan accordingly.

FITNESS TO GO: YOUR SHOULDERS AND ARMS

Shoulder pain and irritation or tears of your rotator cuff (the muscles that make your shoulders stable) are very common after 40. We never think about our shoulders until they are keeping us up at night, and then they are all we can think about. The problem is that when most of us go to the gym, we work only those big cosmetic muscles we can see—the biceps, triceps, and chest. While these are great to look at, they are not the key players in shoulder health or sports.

A few simple exercises can mean the difference between painless, strong shoulders and agonizing shoulder pain. These are the exercises you need when you are recovering from rotator cuff pain, so keep them handy. You can perform these exercises with exercise bands or light dumbbells. The resistance should be enough that you feel a slight burn in your muscles but not more.

Remember that you want to use only your shoulders for this series of exercises. If you find yourself using your whole back to pull the band or lift the weight, then you are using too much resistance. You will know you are using your back and trunk if they move or jerk when you are lifting your arm.

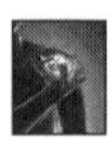 Rotator Cuff Raises (Lateral, Forward, and Across-the-Body)

This set of exercises is the best way to strengthen and maintain the four small but vital muscles of the rotator cuff (supraspinatus, infraspinatus, subscapularis, and teres minor). It should be

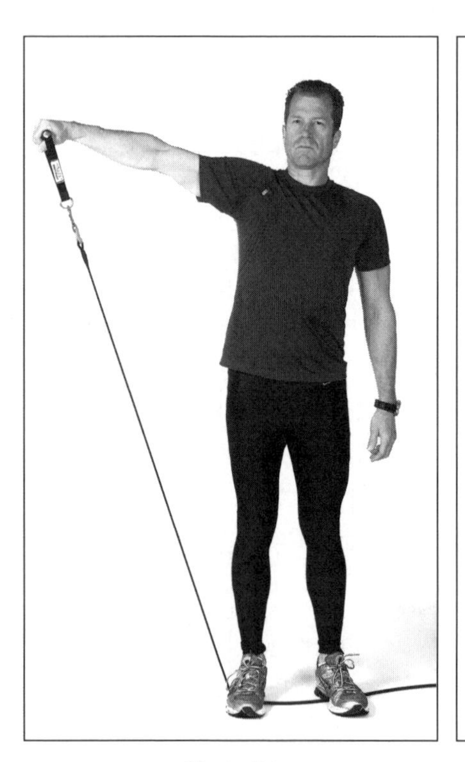

Photo 31

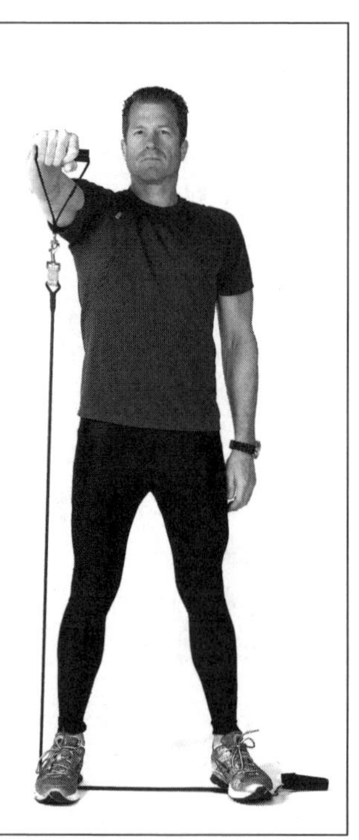

Photo 32

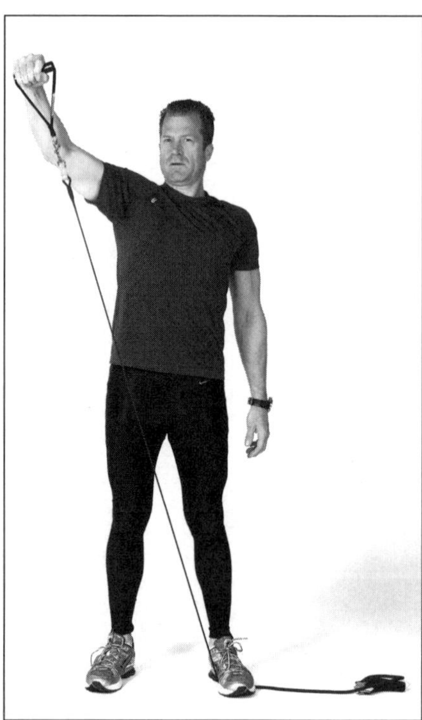

Photo 33

executed in three directions: lateral, forward, and across-the-body.

1. Stand with your feet shoulder-width apart. Engage your core (every exercise can be a core exercise). Place one end of an exercise band under your right foot, and hold the opposite end with your right hand. Slowly raise your right arm to the side until it is level with your shoulder (as shown in Photo 31). Hold for five seconds. Slowly lower your arm. Repeat this nine times to complete one set of Lateral Rotator Cuff Raises.
2. Raise your arm again, this time in front of you (as shown in Photo 32). Be aware of your back. You should be using only your shoulder to raise the band and not leaning backward to raise your arm. Hold for five seconds, then lower your arm slowly. Repeat nine times to complete one set of Forward Rotator Cuff Raises.
3. Place the band under your left foot and continue to hold the band with your right hand. Raise your right arm across your body in a V motion until it is parallel with your shoulder (as shown in Photo 33). Hold for five seconds, then slowly lower your arm. Repeat nine times to complete one set of Across-the-Body Rotator Cuff Raises.
4. Repeat each of these three exercises with the band in your left hand.

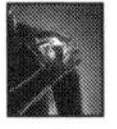 External and Internal Rotation

These exercises work the infraspinatus and subscapularis muscles.

1. Place one end of an exercise band around a sturdy object, such as a doorknob, and stand with your left side toward the

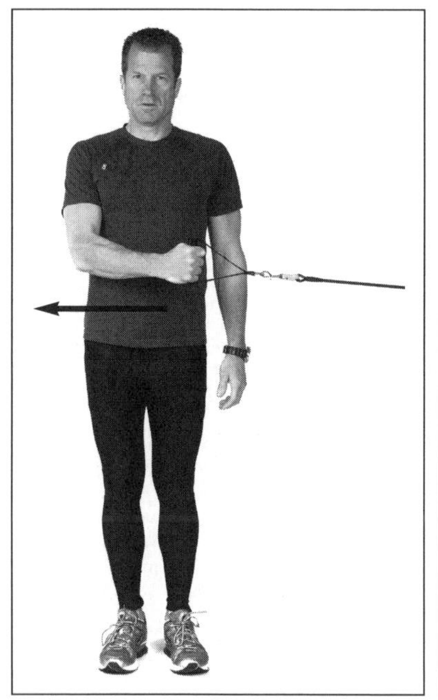

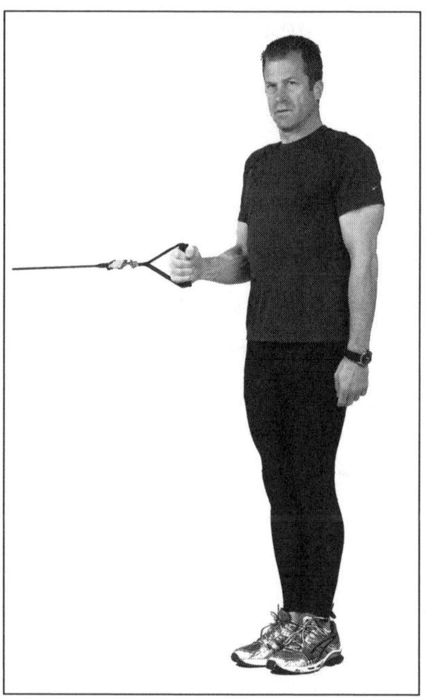

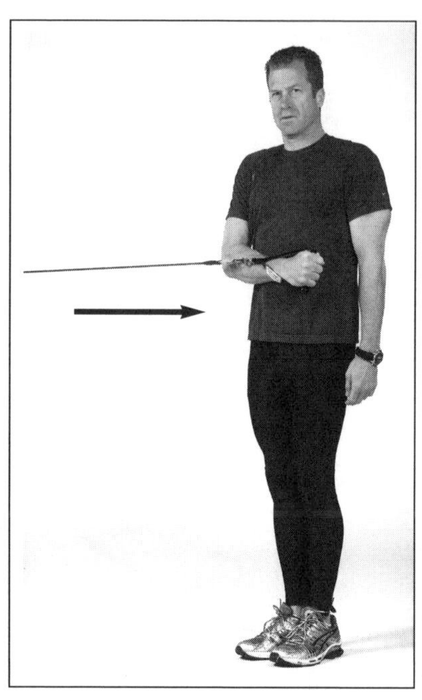

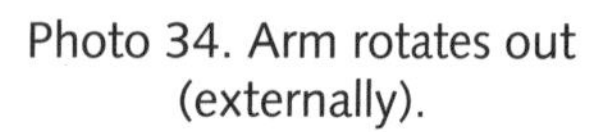

Photo 34. Arm rotates out (externally).

Photo 35

Photo 36. Arm rotates in (internally, across the body).

door. Hold the other end of the band in your right hand (as shown in Photo 34).

2. Pull the band away from your body with your elbow against your left side. Repeat this nine times to complete one set of External Rotations.
3. With the exercise band still tied to a sturdy object such as a doorknob, stand facing the door (as shown in Photo 35). Pull the band across your body with your right elbow against your right side (as shown in Photo 36). Repeat this nine times to complete one set of Internal Rotations.
4. Adjust your body in relation to the door as needed and repeat both exercises with the left arm.

Kettle Bell Shrug

Your shoulder health is related to the strength of your trapezius and upper back. This exercise works these muscles while engaging your shoulders and core.

1. Place your feet slightly wider than shoulder-width apart. Hold a kettle bell in your right hand in front of your body at arm's length.
2. Lower into a half squat with hips pushed back and knees bent 60 degrees (as shown in Photo 37).
3. Thrust your hips forward while simultaneously squeezing your butt together, allowing your knees to straighten to a

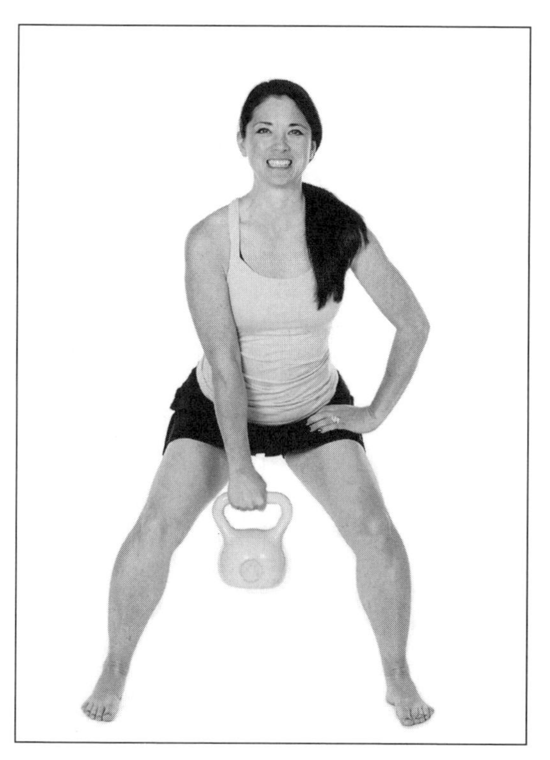

Photo 37

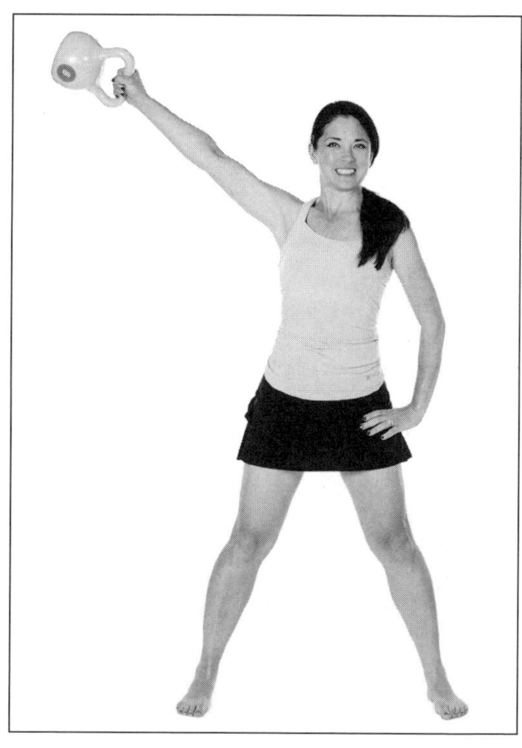

Photo 38

standing position, and swinging the kettle bell up to chest level, or, if possible, above your head (as shown in Photo 38).

4. Return to a squat position as you swing the kettle bell down between your legs. Repeat nine times to complete one set.
5. Switch the kettle bell to the left hand and repeat Steps 1–4.

Biceps Curl

Ahhh, the "guns." No explanation is needed, as you strengthen the key muscles for lifting objects toward your head and pulling things toward you. Plus they look great!

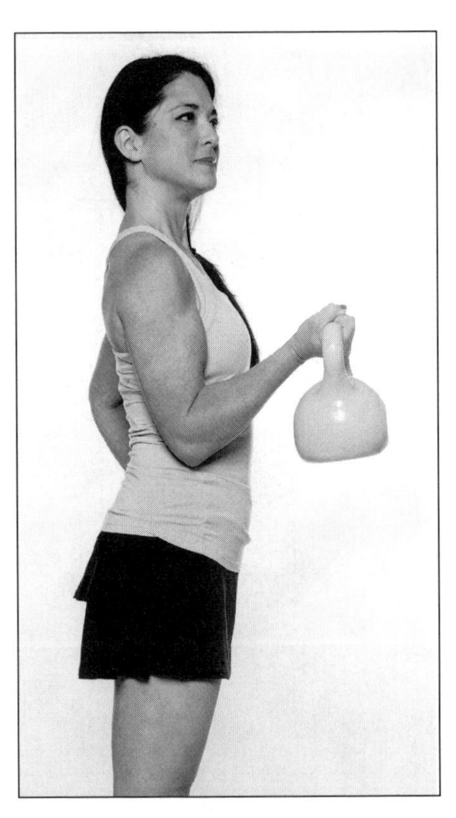

Photo 39

1. While holding a free weight or kettle bell in your right hand, stand with your feet shoulder-width apart and brace your core.
2. Turn your right palm forward.
3. Keep your right elbow next to your body and your upper arm still. Bend your elbow to curl the weight up toward your shoulders (as shown in Photo 39), then slowly lower the weight back to your starting position.
4. Repeat Step 3 nine times to complete one set.
5. Switch the free weight or kettle bell to your left hand and repeat Steps 1–4.

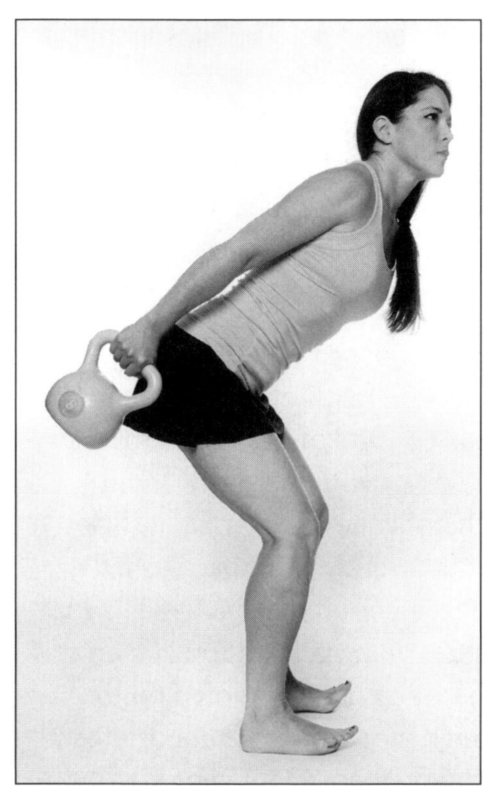

Photo 40

Triceps Extension

You need to balance every muscle group—and the triceps balance the biceps.

1. Stand with your feet shoulder-width apart and knees bent while holding a free weight or kettle bell in your right hand.
2. Engage your core and bend forward at the waist, keeping your back straight.
3. Keeping your right elbow close to your side, bend your arm and lift the weight toward your chest.
4. To fire your triceps, extend your arm to a straightened position (as shown in Photo 40) and hold the position for three seconds. Then, slowly flex your biceps to return to the starting position.
5. Repeat Steps 2–4 nine times to complete one set, then switch the free weight or kettle bell to your left hand and repeat.

FITNESS TO GO: YOUR LOWER BACK AND CORE

The key to your back is your front. The muscles of the lower back are actually smaller than the muscles of the abdomen and sides. The large rectus muscles in the front and the oblique muscles on your sides—also known as your core—stabilize your back and pelvis and, if strong, act to prevent pain. The most important way to prevent lower back pain and the misery it causes is to concentrate on your core muscles. Core strength is also vital for all sports from running (runners notoriously have weak core strength) to golf (how do you think Tiger Woods drives the ball so far?). No matter what your sport, if you have a weak core, this is only because you do not specifically pay attention to it.

We've mentioned the core a number of times, but what exactly is your core? Your core is the "belt" of muscles that wraps around your midsection. It consists of the rectus muscles, which give you the "six pack" look of your stomach. More importantly, it also consists of the oblique or diagonal muscles, which wrap around the sides of your body from back to front, forming a natural weight belt. Place your hands just above your hips and tighten the muscles under your palms. (You can do this not by sucking in your stomach but by pushing down on the pelvis with your muscles. Although indelicate, it is almost like pushing down to have a bowel movement.) Engaging this natural weight belt is called "bracing." Once you start bracing these muscles frequently, you will notice them getting tighter. If you can't feel them getting tight now, it does not mean they are not there; they just have not been engaged in a long time. Your goal is to keep these muscles working throughout the day, even when you are not exercising.

You should perform the following exercises at least three days a week. Do them while relaxing after work. If you can do only one of the exercises, choose the Plank.

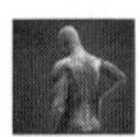 Dying Bug

This exercise stabilizes your lower core and hip flexors.

1. While lying on your back, raise your left arm over your head and bend your right knee to 90 degrees.

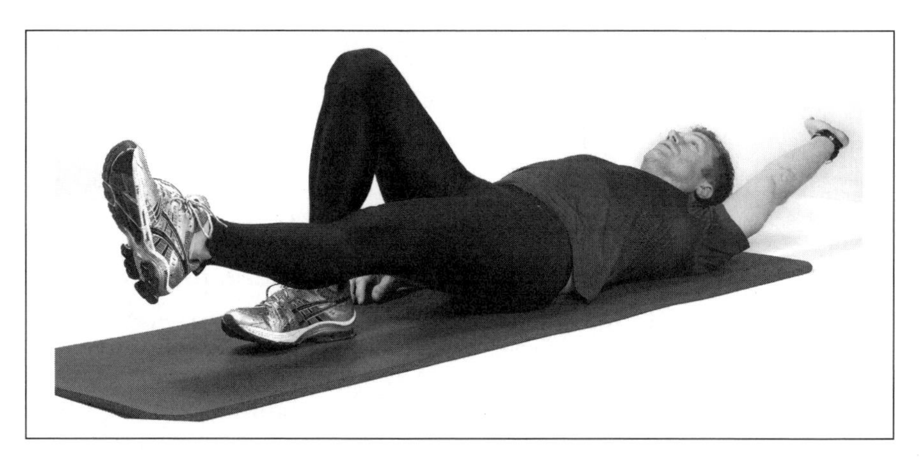

Photo 41

2. Brace your core muscles.
3. Without swaying your back, raise your left leg up off the floor approximately 12 inches and hold for a count of three (as shown in Photo 41). Then lower your left leg.
4. Repeat Steps 1–3 nine times to complete one set, then change arms and legs.

Plank

My personal favorite, this exercise is great for your whole core. You will feel it in your lower core muscles.

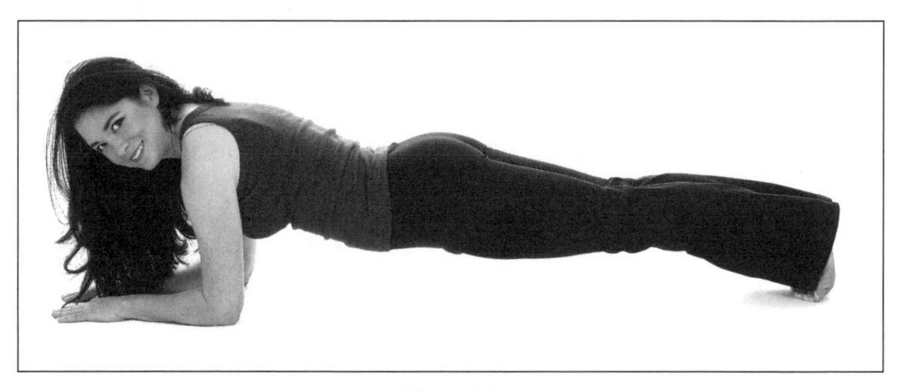

Photo 42

1. Lie down on your stomach and brace your core muscles.
2. Raise your body up on your toes and elbows. To protect your shoulders, make sure they are directly over your elbows (and not forward).
3. Lower your buttocks until they are level with your shoulders (as shown in Photo 42). Squeeze your navel toward your spine. This is the key to this exercise and really works the core.
4. Hold for 30 seconds. (Alternatively, you can hold for 10 seconds and repeat nine times to complete one set.) As you improve, you can increase the hold to two minutes.

Note: If you find it difficult to do the Plank while resting on your toes (as you may if your upper body is not strong enough to hold you up), you can still work your core by balancing on your knees instead. When your core and upper body strength increases, you can switch to doing the Plank while resting on your toes.

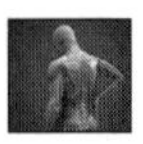 Side Plank

Another favorite, this exercise is key for strengthening your obliques and whittling away your waist.

1. Lie on your left side and brace your core muscles.
2. Raise your trunk off the floor, supporting your weight on your left foot and your left forearm (as shown in Photo 43). Do not let your middle sag. Make sure your shoulder is directly over your elbow.
3. Squeeze your obliques. (The obliques, which are the muscles that cover the sides of your body, were discussed previously in this chapter.)

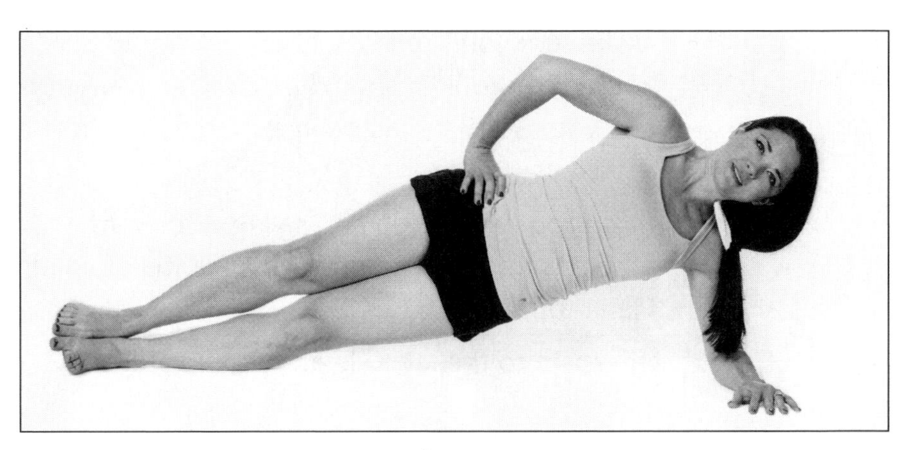

Photo 43

4. Hold for 30 seconds. (Alternatively, you can hold for 10 seconds and repeat nine times to complete one set.) As you improve, you can increase the hold to two minutes.
5. Switch to your right side and repeat Steps 1–4.

Note: If your upper body is not strong enough at this point to support you as you balance on your forearm and foot, bend your knees and rest the weight of your lower body on them. When your core and upper body strength increases, you can switch to doing the Side Plank while resting on your foot.

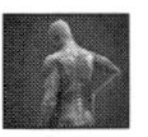 Side Plank with Upper Leg Swing

Once the Side Plank is easy for you, increase the work by adding motion. This forces dynamic stabilization of your core and pelvis.

1. Lie on your right side and engage your core and squeeze your butt.
2. Raise your trunk off the floor, supporting your weight on your right foot and your right forearm (as shown in Photo 44).

Make sure your butt is neither sticking up nor sinking down. Your right shoulder should be directly over your right elbow and your body should be in a straight line from ankles to shoulders.

3. Raise your left leg up and swing it forward and backward 10 times to complete one set while maintaining great Side Plank form.
4. Alternate to the left side and repeat Steps 1–3.

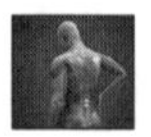 Side Plank with Upper Leg Lift

Side Plank experts will enjoy this variation as well, as it forces engagement of the opposite side obliques.

1. Lie on your right side and engage your core and squeeze your butt.
2. Raise your trunk off the floor, supporting your weight on your right foot and your right forearm (as shown in Photo 44). Make sure your butt is neither sticking up nor sinking

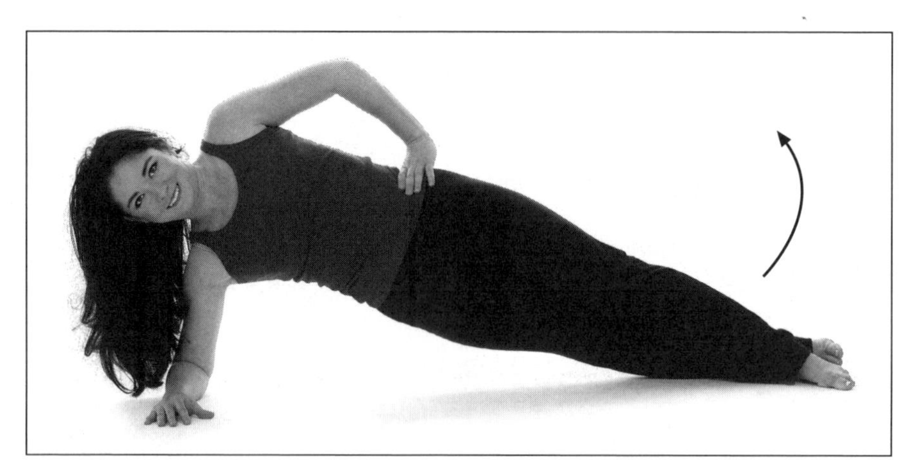

Photo 44

down. Your right shoulder should be directly over your right elbow and your body should be in a straight line from ankles to shoulders.

3. Raise your left leg up as high as you can and hold it for up to 45 seconds. Lower your leg, then repeat nine times to complete one set.
4. Alternate to the left side and repeat Steps 1–3.

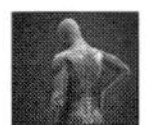 Superman (and Woman!)

You have a front core and a back core. This exercise strengthens the tiny, but important, multifidus muscles in your back.

1. While lying flat on the floor, brace your trunk.
2. Extend your arms above your head.
3. Raise your arms and legs off the floor simultaneously (as shown in Photo 45). Hold for five seconds, then relax.
4. Repeat Step 3 nine times to complete one set.

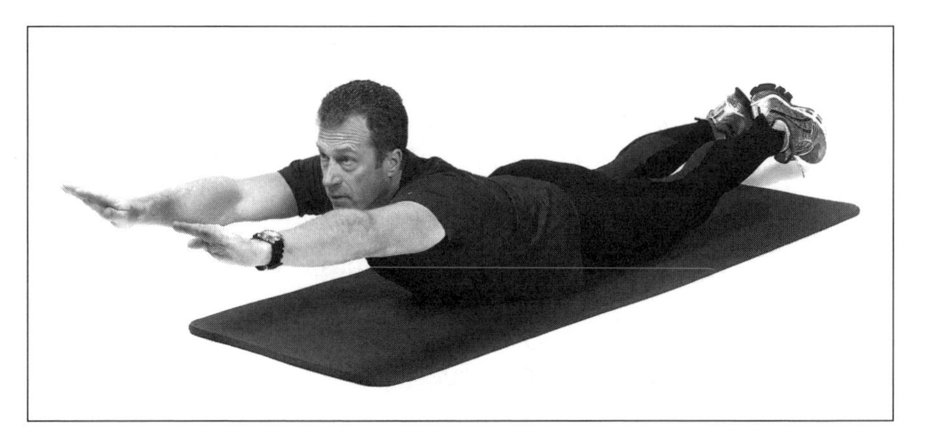

Photo 45

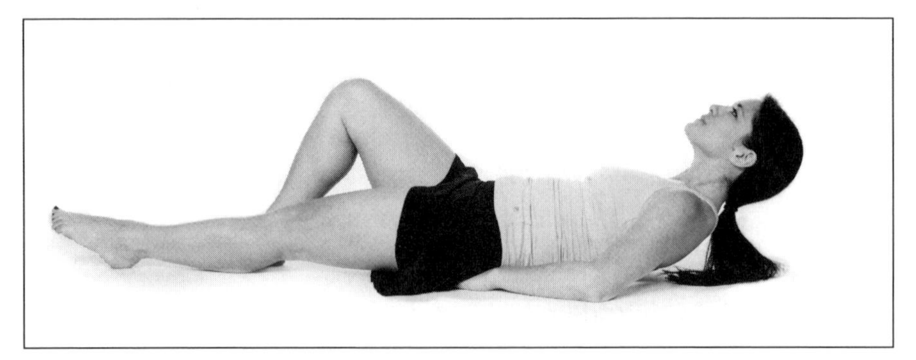

Photo 46

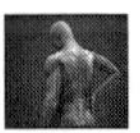 Classic Crunch

As a hip surgeon, I am not crazy about the Classic Crunch because people so often use their hip flexors (instead of their core) to raise their trunks. When doing this exercise, make sure to isolate your core by truly raising your trunk to the ceiling and not simply bending at the waist.

1. Lie flat on the floor, bend one knee to 90 degrees to stabilize your pelvis, and place your arms alongside your body.
2. Engage your core and, keeping your chin pointing forward and exhaling as you go up, raise your head and shoulders off the floor without flexing your lower spine (as shown in Photo 46). Your aim is to move your chest toward the ceiling, not toward your knees.
3. Inhale as you lower your shoulders and head.
4. Repeat Steps 1–3 nine times to complete one set.

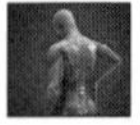 Russian Twist

This core exercise is for people who have mastered the basic moves and are looking for a challenge. It engages the front core, the obliques, and motion all at once.

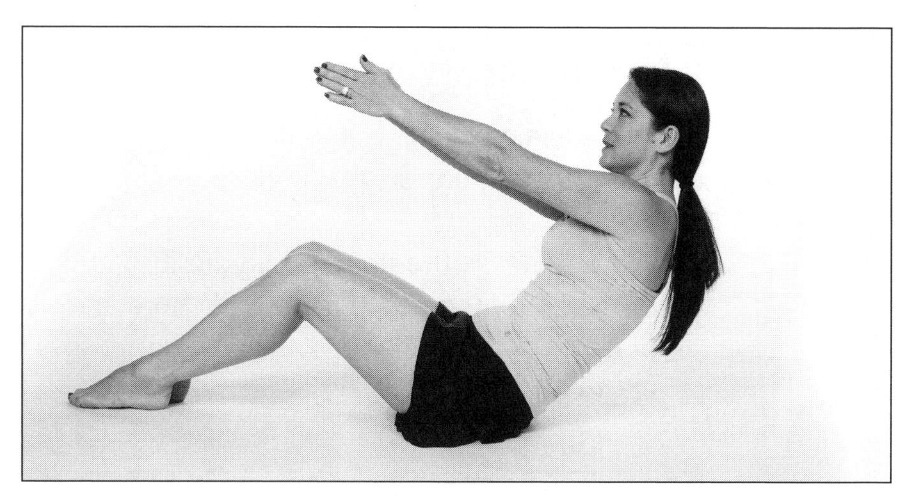

Photo 47

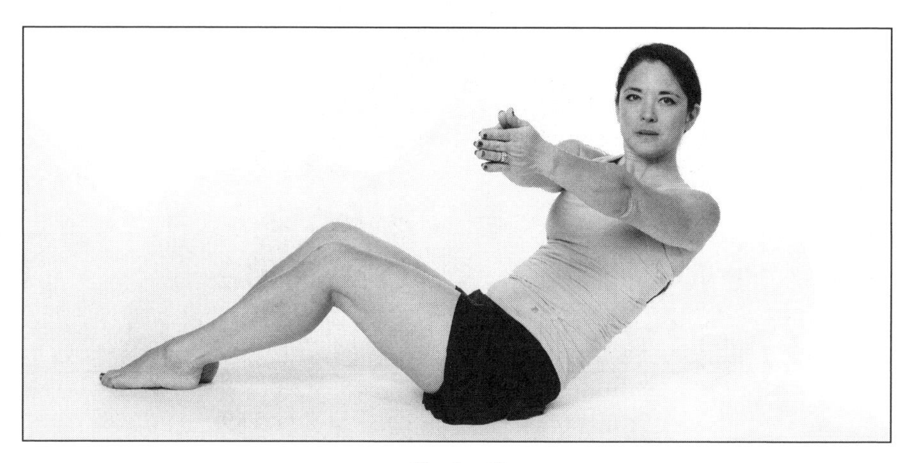

Photo 48

1. Engage your core and sit with your trunk at a 45-degree angle. Bend your knees to 45 degrees and keep your feet flat on the floor.
2. Extend your arms, palms together, in front of your body (as shown in Photo 47).
3. Rotate your arms and trunk to the right as far as you can. Then rotate your arms and trunk to the left as far as you can (as shown in Photo 48).
4. Repeat Step 3 nine times to complete one set.

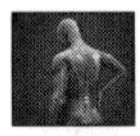 Oblique Twist

This floor-lying exercise is another great variation for your oblique muscle groups.

1. While lying on the floor, raise your legs and bend your knees to 90 degrees. Engage your core and balance your body by extending your arms out to the sides (as shown in Photo 49).

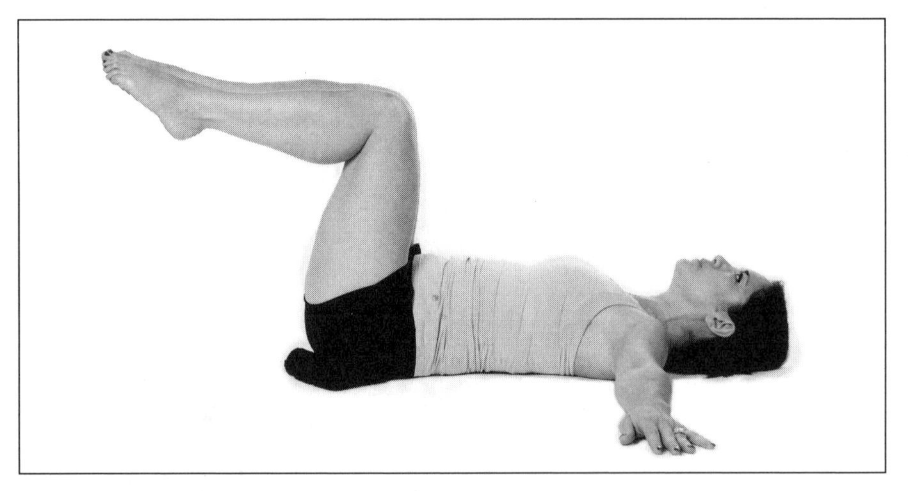

Photo 49

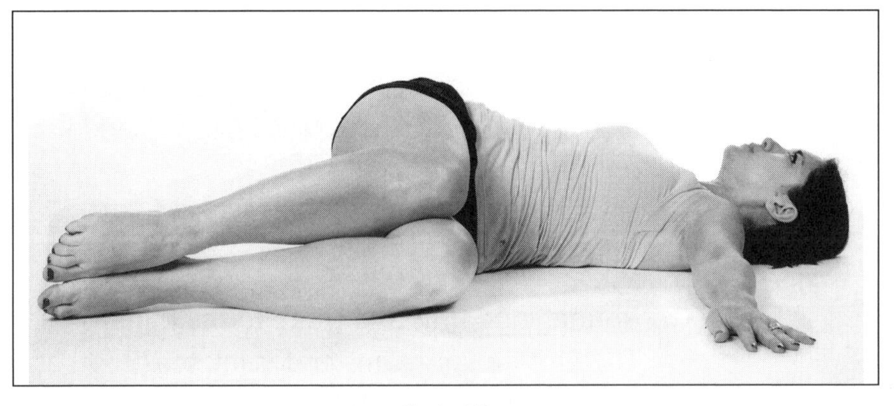

Photo 50

2. Lower your legs to the floor to the right while keeping your shoulders on the floor. You will feel a stretch, but not pain, in your core and lower back.
3. Cross your hips over to the left (as shown in Photo 50), then return to the starting position.
4. Repeat Steps 1–3 nine times to complete one set.

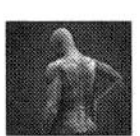 Mountain Climber

This, too, is extra for experts. Form is everything for this exercise, and you may need to use a mirror to ensure that

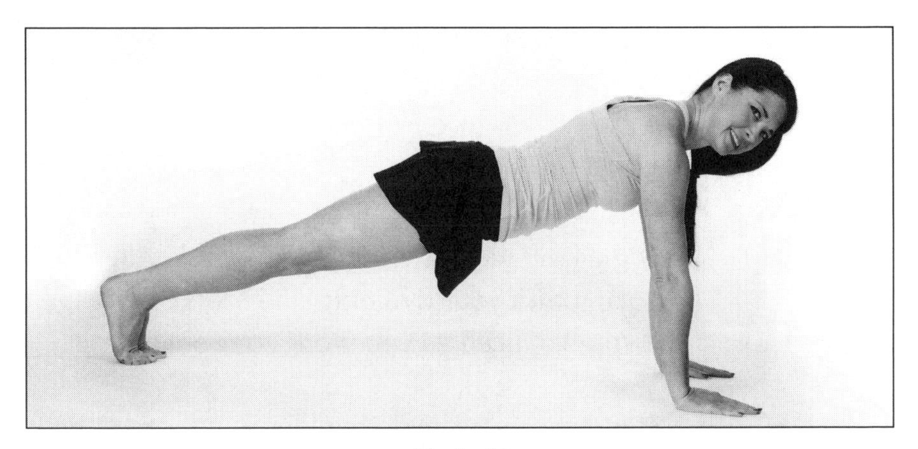

Photo 51

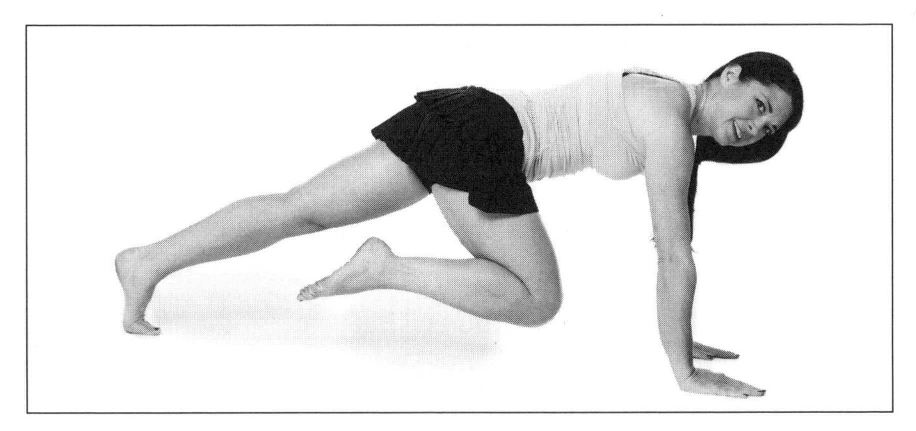

Photo 52

you're employing the best form. Make sure your back is flat as your bring your knee toward your chest.

1. Engage your core and assume a push-up position with your arms straight and your body forming a straight line from shoulders to ankles (as shown in Photo 51).
2. Lift your right foot off the floor and bring your right knee toward your chest as far as you can (as shown in Photo 52), keeping your back straight. Return to the starting position.
3. Alternate legs and bring your left knee toward your chest as far as you can, then return to the starting position.
4. Repeat Steps 2–3 nine times to complete one set.

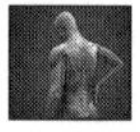 Kettle Bell Twist

Adding a little weight, in the form of a kettle bell (or free weight), forces your dynamic stabilizers to engage even more to keep you balanced as you work your obliques.

1. Stand with your feet shoulder-width apart, with your back straight and your core engaged.
2. Hold a kettle bell (or free weight) in both hands next to your left shoulder (as shown in Photo 53).
3. Bring the kettle bell across the front of your body to the outside of your right knee in a controlled manner by contracting your right oblique muscles (as shown in Photo 54). Pause in this position.
4. Bring the kettle bell back across the front of your body and up to your left shoulder. Repeat nine times to complete one set.

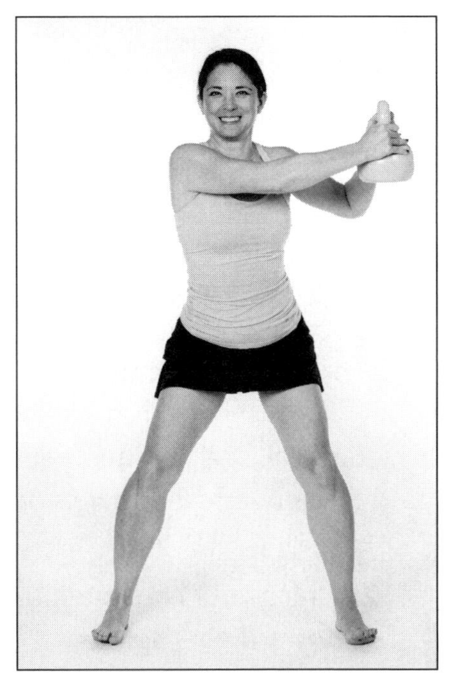

Photo 53

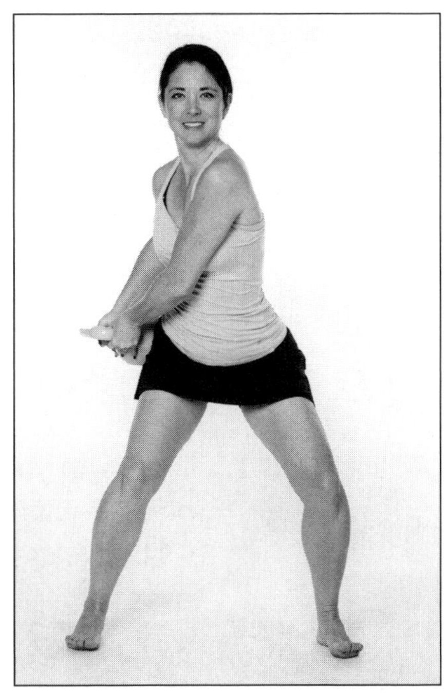

Photo 54

5. Repeat Steps 2–4 on the opposite side, starting with both hands next to your right shoulder and moving to your left knee.

FITNESS TO GO: YOUR BUTT, QUADS, AND KNEES

The keys to almost all activities—including walking, running, climbing, bike riding, and even getting out of a chair—are the muscles of your buttocks (the three layers of gluteus muscles), your core muscles (front and back), and the muscles of your upper legs. Many injuries and much pain can be attributed to weakness of these muscle groups. Purposefully focusing on strengthening these muscles will go a long way toward maximizing your performance and minimizing injury.

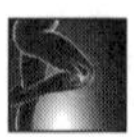 Short Arc Wall Squat

This old faithful can be done at home, work, or any place there is a wall. Try it the next time you are on the phone. This exercise is good for your quadriceps, buttocks, and core.

1. Stand with your back up against a wall and your legs shoulder-width apart. Place two rolled towels or a medicine ball between your knees.

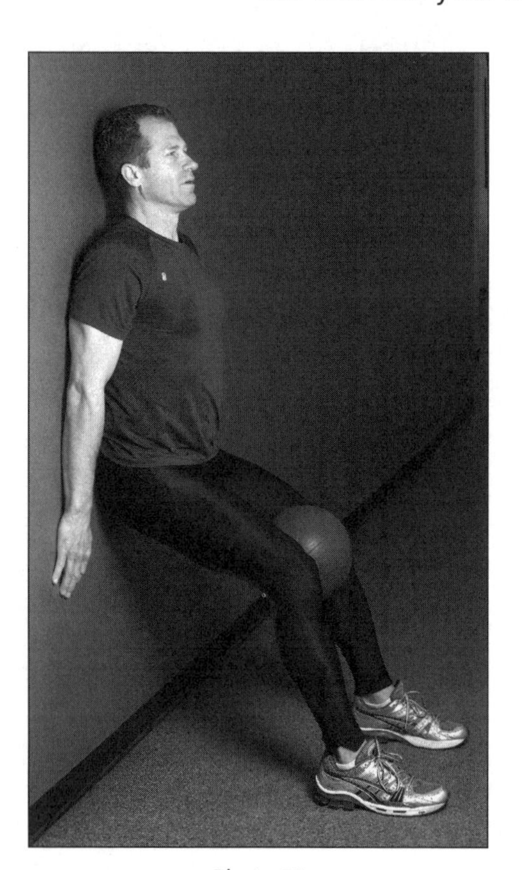

Photo 55

2. Brace your core and pull your navel toward your spine.
3. While keeping your core engaged, slowly slide your back down the wall until your knees are bent to approximately 60 degrees (as shown in Photo 55). This is just shy of parallel to the floor. Limiting the knee bend decreases the pressure on your knees and still works your quads.
4. Hold in the bent position for 10 seconds and then return to a standing position. Repeat nine times to complete one set.

Once you get comfortable doing the Short Arc Wall Squat, you can progress to the more difficult variation, the Prisoner Squat, which appears later in this chapter and is essentially the Short

Arc Wall Squat without the wall. The starting position for a Prisoner Squat features prominently in a number of the exercises toward the end of this chapter.

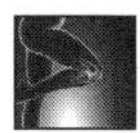 Straight Leg Raise

An old favorite of many trainers (but one of my least favorites), this exercise works the quadriceps, hip flexors, and core. Make sure you are firing and using your quad and not just your hip flexors.

1. Lying flat on your back, engage your core.
2. Bend your right leg up at the knee and keep the left leg straight.
3. Still lying flat on your back, tighten your left quad (front of thigh) and raise your left leg up off the floor until your thighs are parallel. Hold this position five seconds and then lower your leg until it almost touches the floor. Be careful not to let your back sway up off the floor.

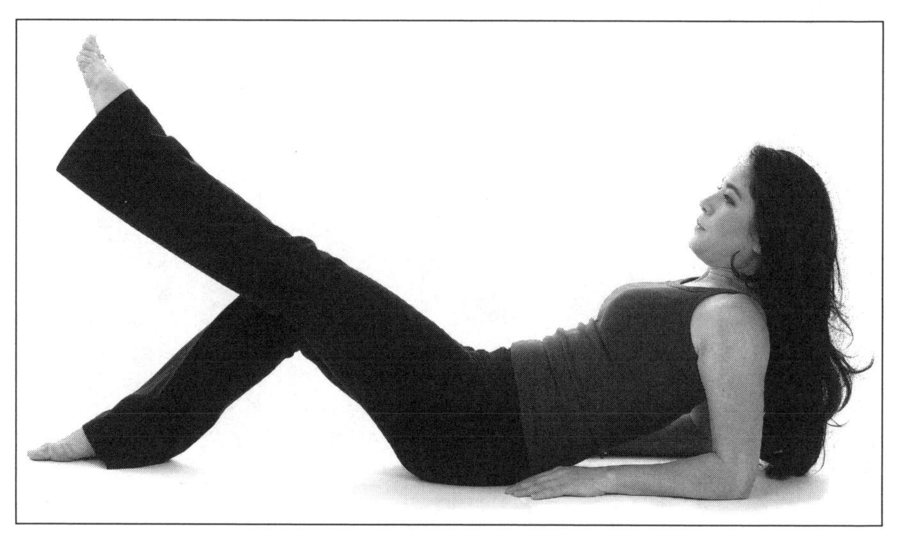

Photo 56

4. Repeat Step 3 nine times to complete one set. Then switch to the right leg.

To increase the difficulty, you can repeat the sets while supporting yourself on your elbows (as shown in Photo 56) or hands.

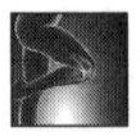 Leg Abduction

This exercise strengthens the muscles that move your leg away from your body's midline.

1. While lying on your left side, brace your abdominal muscles.
2. Bend your left leg forward at the hip and support your trunk with your right arm (as shown in Photo 57).
3. Raise your right leg off the floor and extend behind your body. Do not let your trunk sag backward.
4. Hold for a count of three. Concentrate on keeping your core engaged, and feel this in your buttocks. Return your right leg back to its original position.

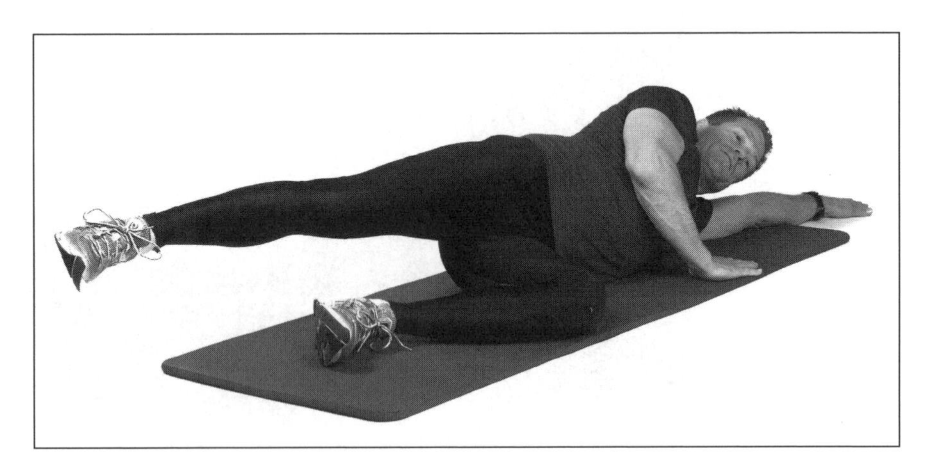

Photo 57

5. Repeat Steps 2–4 nine times to complete one set, then switch to your right side.

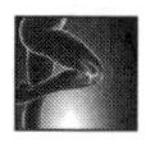 Leg Adduction

This exercise strengthens the muscles that move your leg toward the middle and across your body.

1. While lying on your right side and propping up your chest with your right arm, brace your abdominal muscles.
2. Bend your left knee and place your left foot in front of your right knee.
3. Raise your right leg off the floor (as shown in Photo 58). Do not let your trunk bend backward.
4. Hold for a count of three. Concentrate on keeping your core engaged, and feel this on the inside of your right leg. Lower the right leg back to its original position.
5. Repeat Steps 3–4 nine times to complete one set, then switch to the other side.

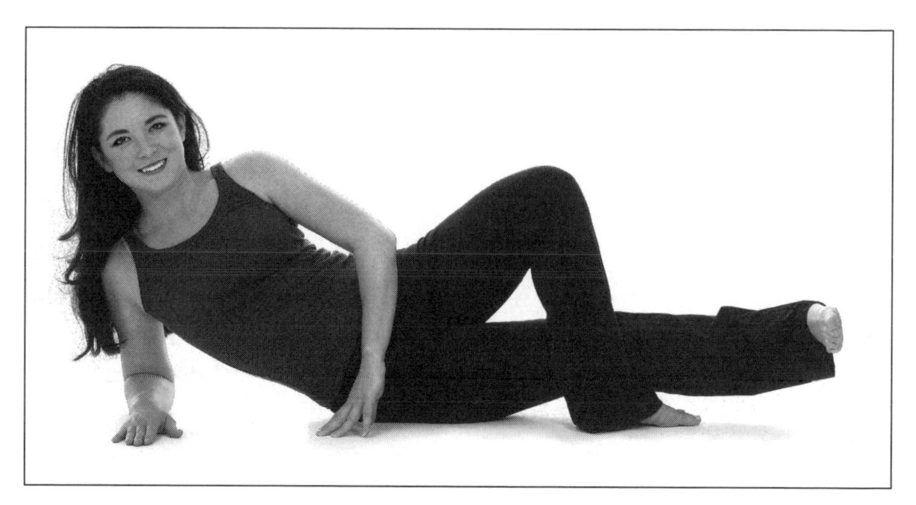

Photo 58

You can combine the Leg Abduction and Leg Adduction exercises. First, do the Leg Abduction. Then, before switching to the other side and without resting, do the Leg Adduction. You can then switch to the other side and begin the Leg Abduction.

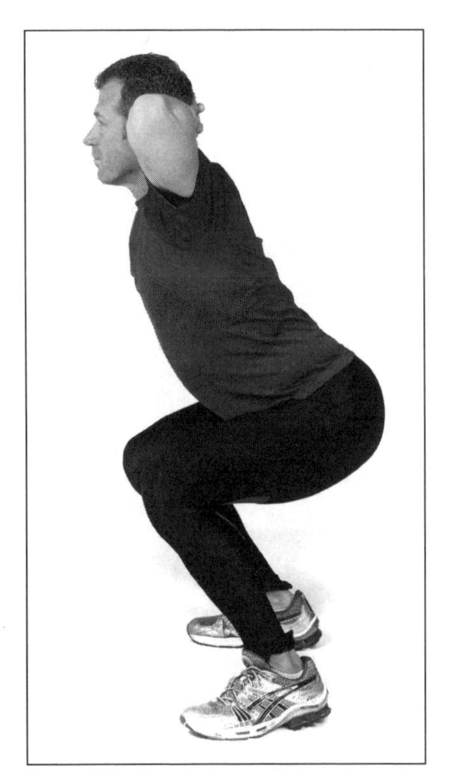

Photo 59

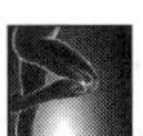 Prisoner Squat

This exercise strengthens your quads, buttocks, and core. It is simply a Short Arc Wall Squat without the wall, which forces you to use your balance to stay upright. Form is important with this exercise. Make sure to lean back so your knees stay above (and not in front of) your ankles.

1. Stand with your feet a little farther than shoulder-width apart and squat down with your knees above your ankles.
2. Keep your back straight and your head up. Hold your hands behind your head (as shown in Photo 59). Then return to a standing position.
3. Repeat Steps 1–2 nine times to complete one set. Try doing one set several times a day.

You can work an upper body workout into the Prisoner Squat by standing with both feet on an exercise band and holding one end in each hand. As you do the squat, pull the band up to your shoulders. If your palms face forward and you pull the band above your shoulders, you will work your back. Alternatively, if your palms face toward you and you keep your elbows in, you can curl your biceps.

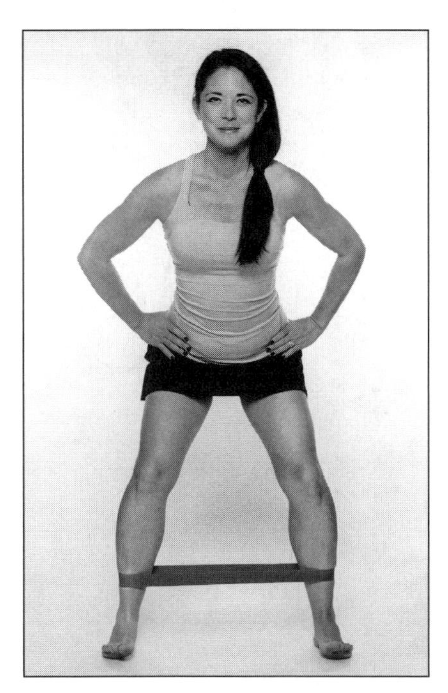
Photo 60

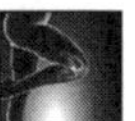 Monster Walk

Nothing is better for isolating your very important gluteus medius muscle than this exercise. It burns like crazy—and is a lot of fun.

1. Place a resistance tube or continuous exercise band just above your ankles.

2. Place your hands on your hips and stand with your feet approximately shoulder-width apart so that there is a gentle tension on the band. Slightly bend your knees and hips (as shown in Photo 60). Engage your core.

3. Take a half step to the side with your right foot and then follow with a half step toward the right foot with your left. Maintain tension on the band at all times and feel the burn in the top of your buttocks.

4. Continue with nine more half steps to the right, and then reverse and take 10 half steps to the left to complete one set. Or simply walk around the room for 45 seconds.

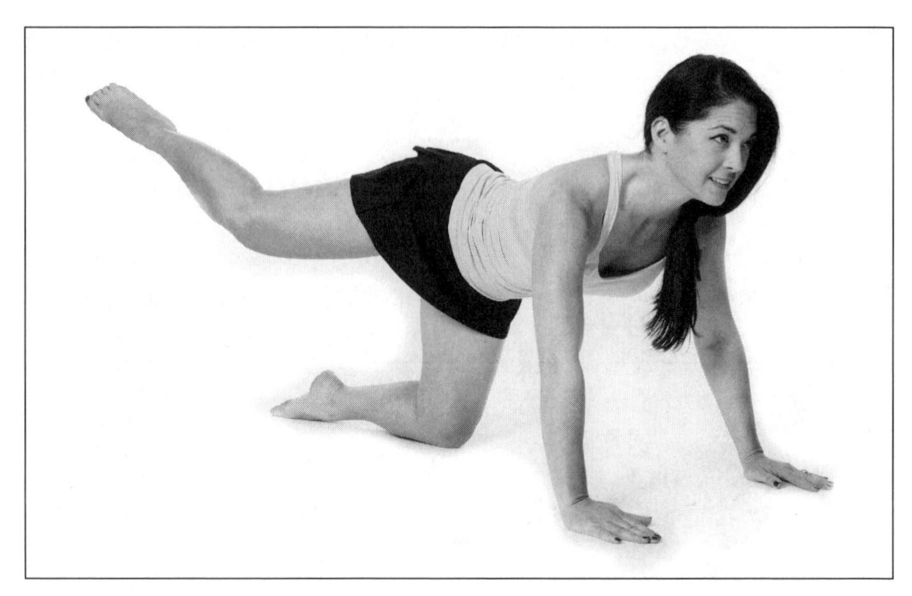

Photo 61

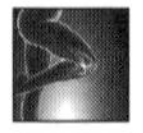 Fire Hydrant

This exercise looks awkward, but it's great for your butt. You will feel the burn if you keep your hips aligned with your knees.

1. Begin on your hands and knees with your hips directly over your knees and your shoulders directly over your hands. Your hands and knees should be shoulder-width apart. Engage your core.
2. Keeping your back straight, raise your right leg to the side with your knee bent. Keep your support (left) hip directly over your left knee.
3. Straighten your right leg back until it is in line with your trunk (as shown in Photo 61), then return to your starting position.
4. Repeat Steps 2–3 nine times to complete one set, then switch to your left leg.

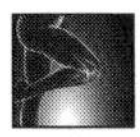 Runner's Lunge

This lunge is important for building your power and neuromuscular control, which allows you to push off with every step you take—whether running or walking.

1. Stand with your left foot in front of your right in a staggered manner with your left knee slightly bent. Your weight should be on the heel of your left foot and the toes of your right.
2. Engage your core and squeeze your butt.
3. Slowly lower your body until your hips are parallel to your left knee. Your left knee should be over your ankle and the right knee should be nearly touching the floor (as shown in Photo 62). Keep your torso upright.
4. Pause in this position while squeezing your butt and pushing your hips slightly forward. Return to the starting position quickly and repeat nine times to complete one set.
5. Switch positions so your right leg is in front of your left and repeat Steps 2–4.

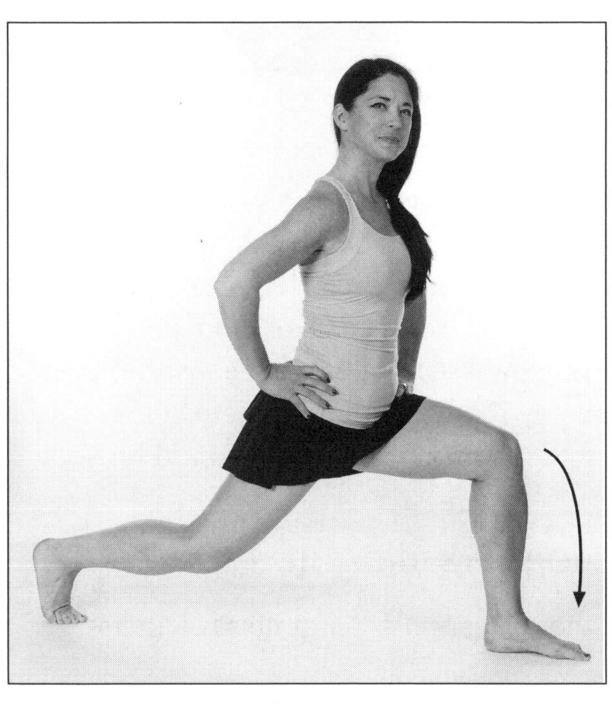

Photo 62

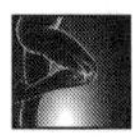 Reverse Split Squat

Although you may think you are doing just another lunge, moving in the reverse direction with your leg forces the front of your body to engage for stability.

1. Stand with your feet together and engage your core.
2. Lunge back with your right foot, while keeping your weight on your left heel (you end in the same position as shown in Photo 62).
3. Tuck your right buttocks under and feel the lengthening of your hip flexor. Hold this lowered position for three seconds, rise out of the lunge, and begin again.
4. Repeat the lowering and rising sequence nine times to complete one set. Then switch to the left foot and repeat.

FITNESS TO GO: YOUR LOWER LEGS

You may not even notice the muscles in the lower part of your legs—that is, until one of them is irritated or inflamed. Weakness in the lower legs can mean pain with each step or sport-halting injury. Shin splints, calf pulls, Achilles tendinitis, and peroneal tendinitis (behind the outer ankles) can be avoided with these simple exercises. If you pay some attention to them, it is easy to keep these forgotten muscles happy and working hard for you.

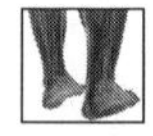 Plantar Flexion/Dorsiflexion

These exercises work the calves and anterior tibialis muscles.

1. Sit on the floor and place a rolled up towel under your ankle and lower calf, if desired.

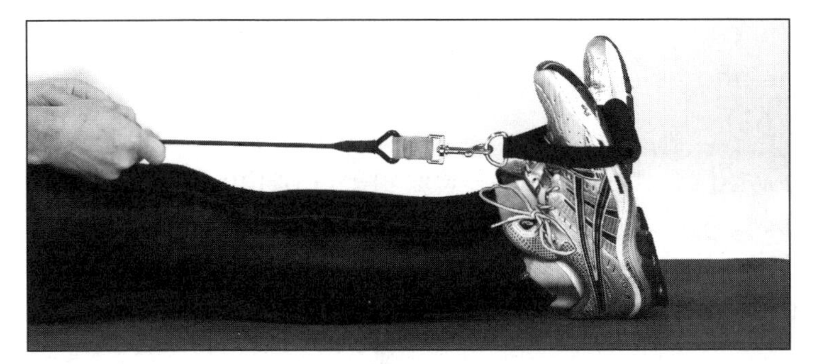

Photo 63

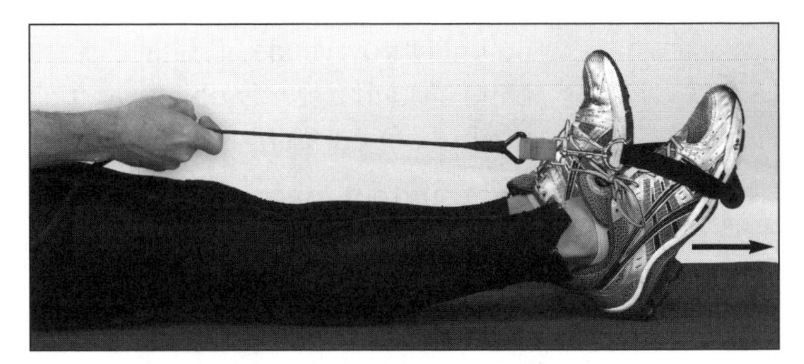

Photo 64. Foot presses forward.

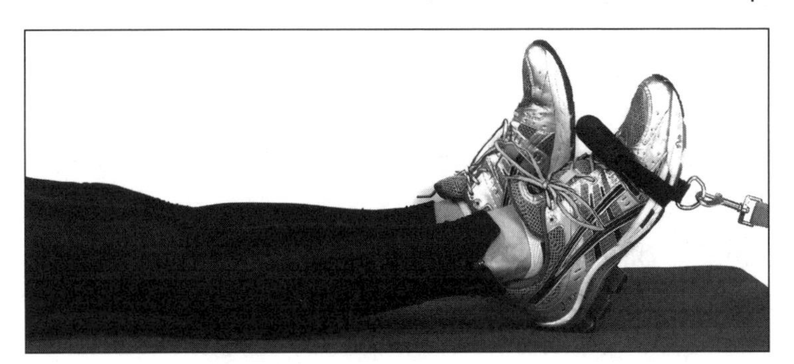

Photo 65

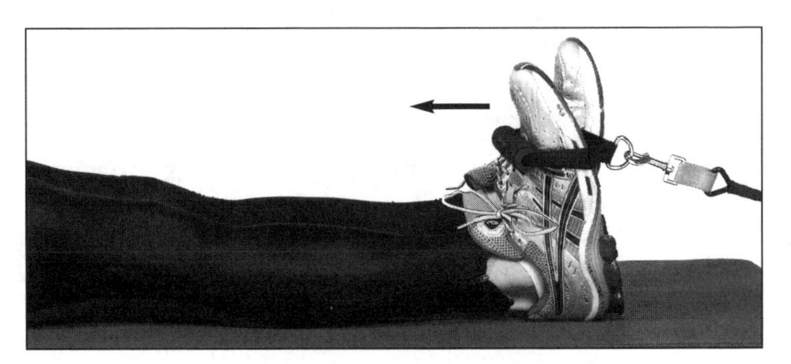

Photo 66. Foot pulls back.

2. Secure the end of an exercise band around the ball of your right foot, and hold the other end with your hands (as shown in Photo 63).
3. Press forward on the band like you are stepping on the gas pedal of your car (as shown in Photo 64). Hold for five seconds. Repeat until your calf (plantar flexion) is fatigued. Switch to your left foot and repeat.
4. To work the front of your legs or your anterior tibialis muscle (dorsiflexion), remain sitting on the floor with a towel rolled up under your ankle, if desired. Secure one end of the exercise band around a sturdy object, and place the other end around the ball of your right foot (as shown in Photo 65).
5. Pull your foot toward your body (as shown in Photo 66). Hold for five seconds. Repeat until the anterior tibialis muscle is fatigued. Switch to your left foot and repeat.

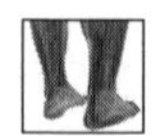 Ankle Inversion/Ankle Eversion

These exercises work the peroneal and posterior tibialis muscles.

1. Sit on the floor and place a rolled-up towel under your ankle and lower calf.
2. Secure one end of an exercise band to a sturdy object and the other end around the ball of your left foot. The band should be stretching away from your body (as shown in Photo 67).
3. Using only your foot and ankle, not your whole leg, pull the band in toward the midline of your body (as shown in Photo 68). Hold for five seconds. Repeat this until fatigue sets in with your posterior tibialis muscles.
4. Keeping the band on your left foot, change positions so that the band is stretching in front of your body.

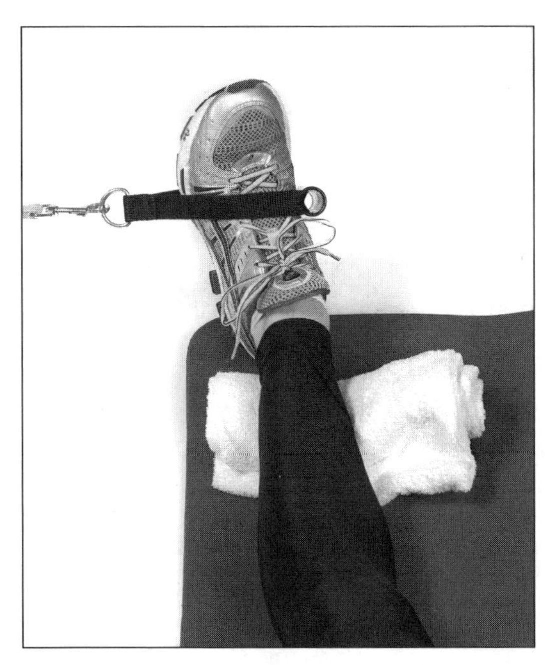

Photo 67

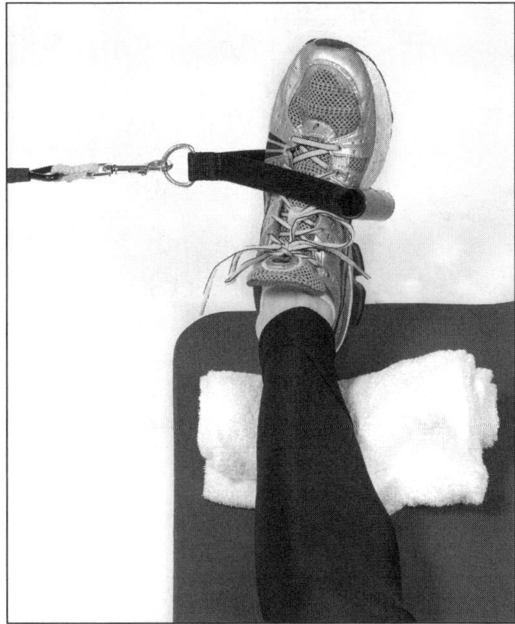

Photo 68. Foot moves in.

5. Using only your foot and ankle, not your whole leg, evert or pull the band so that your foot moves out away from the midline of your body. Hold your foot everted for five seconds, and repeat until fatigue sets in with your peroneal muscles.
6. Move the band to your right foot and repeat Steps 2–5, adjusting the position of the band as necessary.

Even though these leg-strengthening exercises use exercise bands, you can strengthen your lower legs (and prevent muscle imbalance and shin splints) without any equipment at all. The goal is to strengthen the muscles that dorsiflex (bring up) and plantarflex (lower) your ankles. You can do the exercises that follow in your office, at the airport, or in the kitchen while cooking.

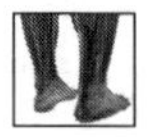 Wall Shin Raise

This exercise works the anterior tibialis muscle in the front of your shin.

1. Stand with your back and shoulders against the wall, with your feet shoulder-width apart and about one foot from the wall.
2. Raise the toes on both your feet simultaneously as high off the ground toward your body as you can with your weight on your heels.
3. Slowly lower your toes until they are almost but not quite on the floor, and then flex them up again. Repeat this nine times to complete one set.

As you get better at this exercise, you can "pulse" quickly from flexing up to extending your ankle down. Once you can comfortably complete the Wall Shin Raise (both basic and quick), progress to the Single-Leg Wall Shin Raise. The basic position for this exercise is the same as for the double-leg raise, except that you begin with only one foot in contact with the ground and the other foot resting lightly on the wall behind you. Now, as you carry out the overall routine, your full body weight is on one foot, as it is during running, and the exercises are considerably more difficult.

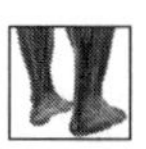 Heel Step Down

This is a great exercise for preventing shin splints.

1. Stand with your feet together and take a natural step forward with your right foot.

2. As your heel strikes the floor, prevent your right foot from flexing down as you transfer your weight forward. This forces your anterior tibialis muscles to contract and mimics the foot action during running.
3. Shift your weight backward and return your right foot to the starting position. Repeat nine times to complete one set.
4. Switch to the left foot and repeat Steps 1–3.

When you have mastered this with short strides, increase your stride length to make the exercise more difficult.

FITNESS TO GO: YOUR WHOLE BODY POWER

Nobody moves only one muscle at a time. This is especially true when you are moving dynamically from one place to another—in life or in exercise. The exercises in this section force the muscles you are building to coordinate with one another and act together for speed, power, and agility. These exercises are all the assets you need for maximizing performance and minimizing injury after age 40.

Vertical Jump

How high is your vertical leap? Measure it now, and then again after you have invested in carrying a load for six weeks. You will marvel at your increased strength and your power to get off the ground!

1. Keeping your trunk upright, engage your core and lower your body into a Prisoner Squat (this is like a Short Arc Wall Squat,

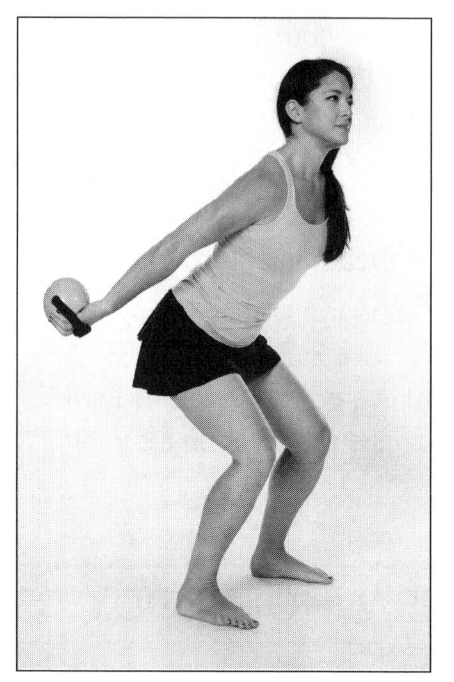

Photo 69

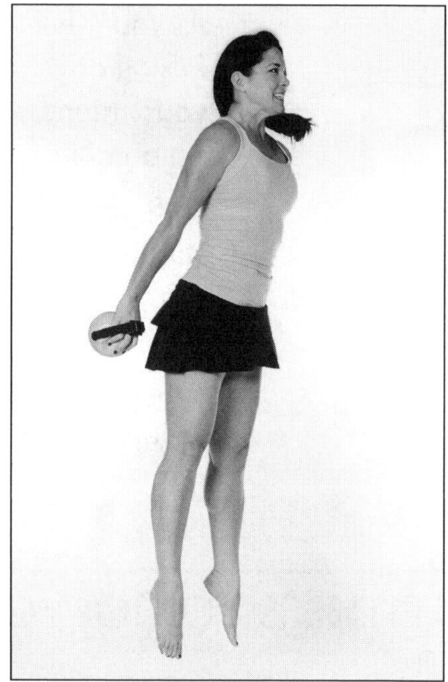

Photo 70

shown previously in this chapter, without the wall) with your butt, back, and knees over your ankles and your feet shoulder-width apart. You may hold small weights, yoga balls, or kettle bells in your hands to add a level of difficulty (as shown in Photo 69).

2. Jump as high in the air as you can, keeping your arms by your side (as shown in Photo 70).
3. Land on the ground with your knees bent and your feet shoulder-width apart. Take care to land with your knees over your ankles (and not over your toes) in order to prevent pain in the front of your knees.

4. Maintain/regain your balance and repeat Steps 1–3 nine times to complete one set.

Plyo Jump

Building explosive strength incorporates your butt, core, and leg muscles, plus balance—all at the same time. (By the way, *plyo* is short for "plyometrics," which is an exercise that involves rapid stretching and contracting of muscles to increase muscle power.)

1. Keeping your trunk upright, engage your core and lower your body into a Reverse Split Squat with your right leg back.
2. Explode up into the air. Switch leg positions midair and land with your left leg back.
3. Maintain/regain your balance and repeat the jump nine times, alternating your lead leg with each jump, to complete one set.

Side Shuffle

Engage your core and use all the lateral muscle groups you just strengthened to perform this fun exercise.

1. Hold a medicine ball in both hands at chest level in front of your body.
2. Assume a Prisoner Squat position, with your butt back and your knees over your ankles, and engage your core.
3. Remain in this squat position while you shuffle your feet to the right for 10 steps and then shuffle back to the left for 10 steps. Do this as rapidly as you can without losing your balance or your form.
4. Repeat this motion two additional times to complete one set.

Grapevine Step

Add a little agility and balance to your life with this move, which you may remember from your school days. Be careful not to trip over your own two feet!

1. Stand with your feet together and engage your core.
2. Step to the right with your right foot and quickly follow with a step to the right with your left foot, landing behind your right.
3. Step to the right with your right foot and quickly follow with a step to the right with your left foot, landing in front of your right.
4. Step to the left with your left foot and quickly follow with a step to the left with your right foot, landing behind your left.
5. Step to the left with your left foot and quickly follow with a step to the left with your right foot, landing in front of your left.
6. Repeat Steps 2–5 as rapidly as possible, swinging your arms front and back for balance, for either 45 seconds or a distance of 20 yards.

Standing Broad Jump

As with the Vertical Jump, the power and distance you display when doing this exercise measures your total body power, as covering a distance takes a strong core, butt, and legs.

1. Assume a Prisoner Squat position with your butt back and your knees over your ankles and engage your core.
2. Swing your arms to propel your body and leap forward.

3. Land in the same Prisoner Squat position.
4. Repeat nine times to complete one set.

Forward Jump and Stick Landing

It is not enough to be strong and powerful if your balance is not in tune. All exercises with "stuck" landings require you to draw upon your balance to stay upright. If you fall over when doing this exercise, work hard on the equilibrium and balance exercises found in Chapter 9.

1. Assume a Prisoner Squat position with your butt back and your knees over your ankles and engage your core.
2. Swing your arms to propel your body and leap forward.
3. Land in a bent knee position on your right foot. Do your best to stick the landing. Regain your balance then lower your left foot to the ground and assume the Prisoner Squat position.
4. Repeat Steps 2–3, this time landing on your left foot.
5. Repeat the sequence nine times to complete one set. Form and balance are more important than speed.

Two-Way Hop (Right and Left)

While I'm not calling this exercise Bunny Hop, you may feel like a rabbit as you hop diagonally and use your lateral stabilizers to stay upright as you build power. This is a variation of the Standing Broad Jump, except that each jump covers a shorter distance (and therefore is a hop) and that you leap in diagonal directions rather than forward.

1. Assume a Prisoner Squat position and engage your core.

2. Swinging your arms to propel your body, hop in a diagonal direction to the right two times. Maintain your balance and keep your knees over your ankles.
3. Still swinging your arms to propel your body, hop in a diagonal direction twice to the left.
4. Repeat the sequence (two hops to the right and two hops to the left) as rapidly as possible with good form nine times to complete one set.

Two-Way Hop (Front and Back)

This is a second variation of the Standing Broad Jump, again with each jump covering a shorter distance.

1. Assume a Prisoner Squat position and engage your core.
2. Swinging your arms to propel your body, hop forward two times. Maintain your balance and keep your knees over your ankles.
3. Switching directions (but not body position), hop backward two times.
4. Repeat the sequence (two hops to the front and two to the back) as rapidly as possible with good form nine times to complete one set.

Triple Jump

This exercise includes three different jumps/hops in a row without stopping. This is a test of your power, agility, and strength.

1. Assume a Prisoner Squat position and engage your core.
2. Beginning on two legs, hop forward and land only on your right foot.

3. Without pausing, hop forward, landing only on your left foot.
4. Without pausing, hop forward again, landing on both feet in the Prisoner Squat position.
5. Repeat Steps 2–4 nine times to complete one set.

Power Skip

This exercise employs exaggerated gestures from your childhood skipping technique. It is fun and powerful.

1. Skip, bringing your knees as high toward your chest as you can and swinging your arms to propel you forward.
2. Continue to skip as fast and as high as you can without falling for 45 seconds or 20 yards to complete one set.

Lateral Hop with Balance

The final exercise in this group puts many skills together, including power from the butt and core and balance from the front and back core. Plus, it engages the lateral stabilizers.

1. Engage your core and slightly bend both of your knees.
2. Look forward and choose a height in front of you to maintain with your eyes. During the hopping sequences that follow, you want to maintain your head height and not bounce up and down.
3. Balance on your left foot and hop quickly to the right, landing on your right foot. Regain your balance on your right foot prior to putting your left foot down.
4. Repeat Step 3 laterally to the right nine times.

5. Change directions. Balance on your right foot and hop to the left, landing on your left foot. Regain your balance on your left foot prior to putting your right foot down.
6. Repeat Step 5 laterally to the left nine times.

HOW TO FIT IT ALL IN

I know I've just given you a lot of new exercises—and this may all seem overwhelming at the moment. To be clear: I am definitely *not* suggesting that you do all of these exercises in one day. What I *do* recommend is that you focus on the "C" (Carry a Load) aspect of F.A.C.E.-ing your future three times a week, and for 20 minutes on each of those three days.

We will discuss various strategies about how to do this in detail in Chapter 10. However, one way that works well for many of my patients is to work on one body part at a time and spread the regimen throughout your day. If you do it this way, it will seem effortless. For instance, you can work your quadriceps before you get out of bed in the morning, work your shoulders while standing in your office talking on the phone, or work your core after your aerobic workout. You can fit it all in because these exercises are fit to go!

At this point, you have a vision of what your physical future can look like, you know how you are different now than you were before, and you are equipped to flex, move, and carry a load. In Chapter 9, you will learn the skill of staying upright.

HOME**WORK**

Carrying a load does not require a big weight machine. All you need to do most of the exercises and circuits in this book is an exercise band, an exercise tube, a kettle bell (or dumbbell), and you! Go to your local sporting goods store today and get prepared.

"Man maintains his balance, poise, and sense of security only as he is moving forward."

—Maxwell Maltz, surgeon and author

CHAPTER NINE 9

E—Equilibrium/ Balance

Don't fall down. Easy advice to give, but in reality—in your forties, fifties, sixties, and beyond—it is not always easy to stay upright. Even if you have not fallen in years, it is likely that you will fall in the future. Did you know that your balance begins to decline after age 25 and that one in three people fall doing normal activities of daily living after age 65? Falls in the later years often result in wrist and hip fractures, which can have a devastating effect on your lifestyle or even threaten your life.

Even if you have mastered the other three components of F.A.C.E.-ing your future, you must never ignore equilibrium and balance, which is an important component of fitness after 40.

Balance is important not only for improving sports performance but even for the mundane activities of life.

SYSTEMS AT WORK

Have you ever stood on the deck of a boat and felt the sway of the water? In order to stay upright, your body is sensing the direction of the sway and activating the muscles on the opposite side of the body to contract and correct your upright position. Your muscles and joints "know" where they are in space. This process, which is called proprioception, happens at lightning speed without your consciously thinking about it. Proprioception is the ability of our bodies to detect where we are in space (i.e., whether we are leaning to the right or left) and to contract muscles appropriately for us to stay upright.

Many systems actually work together to keep us standing upright. Balancing effectively takes our eyes, ears (vestibular system), and peripheral sensory system (skin receptors of pressure and touch) as well as our neuromuscular connections (the nerve pathways among the brain and muscles, tendons, ligaments, and joints). Our brains are able to coordinate these signals to determine where our limbs are in space and the speed and direction of their movement.

With aging, these systems may become less functional, which can lead to imbalance. Our brains miscalculate our position and make errors in determining where our limbs are because the signals our brains receive are less accurate. As our vision and peripheral senses decline, we engage our leg muscles more to prevent sway. To cope, the hip girdle, quadriceps, and muscles surrounding the ankles are engaged to stiffen and freeze the lower legs for upright standing. Since it involves our muscles so much, balance is another reason that maintaining muscle strength is key.

Declines in proprioception and balance are also seen in people who suffer ligament injuries or have osteoarthritis (the "wear-and-tear" type of arthritis). I did a study of Senior Olympians that showed that people with wear-and-tear arthritis of the knee are more likely to have injuries than those who were not diagnosed with arthritis.[1] In addition, we know from multiple studies that if you have arthritis in one knee, not only does your balance decline in that knee but it also declines in the other knee. The reason for this is not clear, but what is clear is that balance and proprioception can be retrained. This is important, since poor balance not only leads to falls but may lead to increased injury.

The good news is that the neuromuscular connections can be entirely reclaimed by specific daily attention. Falls can be prevented. A large analysis of balance studies found that muscle strengthening and balance retraining programs can decrease the risk of falls by 45 percent. In addition, studies show that people who practice the noncompetitive martial art of tai chi (which emphasizes gentle movements and stretching) have a significantly better sense of joint position and better reaction times than people of the same age who did not practice such balance-intense activities.

Aging golfers show the same retention of balance and reaction time as practitioners of tai chi. This makes sense since a good golf swing requires not only balance, with precise control of the head and body in relationship to the legs, but coordinated muscle activity throughout the swing. Overall fitness and lower-extremity muscle strength are important determinants of remaining balanced. Just like any component of fitness, "if you don't use it, you lose it," and—in terms of equilibrium—you can be older than your years.

On the first day of my 12-week PRIMA Start programs, I always talk to our "Starters" about F.A.C.E.-ing their futures and the four components of fitness after 40. They are surprised when I talk about balance and equilibrium. People typically don't realize that their balance is not what it once was until we begin to do some of the warm-up exercises that require standing on one foot. Immediately, their arms are spread out as they try to balance on the ground as if they were on a tightrope wire. We lose our balance subtly, and we don't realize it until we are toppling over. This may be the case for you, too, but it is easy to find out what the state of your neuromuscular connections are.

TEST YOURSELF

You don't have to be falling all around like Jerry's klutzy neighbor Kramer on *Seinfeld* to have a balance problem. Let's test you right now:

1. Stand next to a firm surface such as a counter or chair back.
2. Hold your hands above the surface in case you need support.
3. Close your eyes and lift one foot off the ground.
4. Balance on the other foot.
5. Count out loud the number of seconds you are able to balance.

The shorter your balance time, the "older" your equilibrium is. If you balanced for more than 22 seconds, your balance is as young as a 20-year-old's; 15 seconds, you have the balance of a 30-year-old; 7.2 seconds, of a 40-year-old; 3.7 seconds, of a 50-year-old; and if you toppled over right away, you are 60 in "balance years."

If you are fit and strong, you can have better balance than a much younger sedentary person. There are many ways you can boost your balance.

BALANCE BOOSTERS

The good news is that we can retrain the balance skills we lose with age with these simple balance boosters.

- *Stay strong*. Strengthening your buttocks, quadriceps, and hamstrings go a long way in improving balance.
- *Join a class*. Tai chi, yoga, and Pilates all require slow, deliberate movements, trunk rotation, and one-legged stances.
- *Be productive in your down time*. Between sets of strength exercises, while brushing your teeth in the morning, or while waiting at a street corner for the light to change, try standing on one leg and balancing.
- *Work balance exercises into your daily routine*. You don't need any special equipment—just your body. For best results, do some or all of these exercises every day. It takes four to 12 weeks of work to see a result.

BALANCE EXERCISES

Before beginning any of these exercises, first engage your core muscles. To do this, stand up tall, put your hands on your hips, and bear down until you can feel your core muscles under your hands.

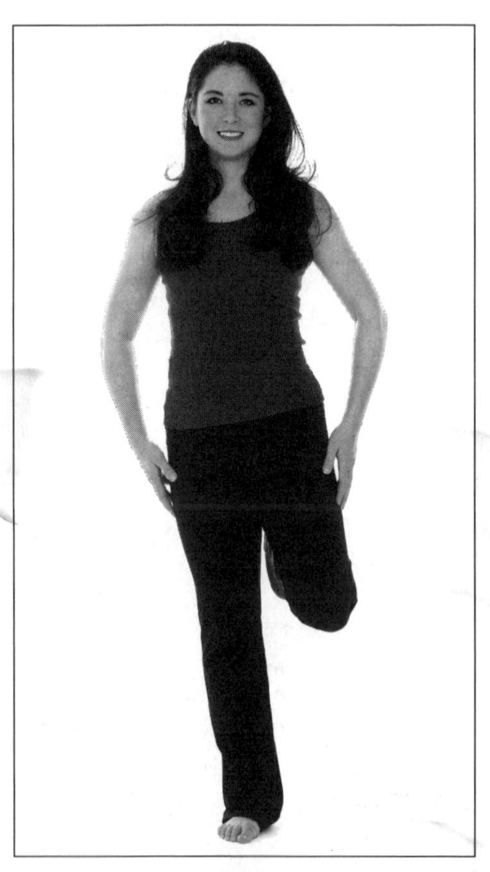

Photo 71

The Stork

This exercise is simple and highly versatile. You can do it while standing anywhere—at the kitchen sink while washing dishes, at your desk while talking on the phone, or in the bathroom while brushing your teeth.

1. Stand with your feet slightly apart and raise your left leg off the ground while keeping your arms to the sides and your shoulders relaxed (as shown in Photo 71).
2. Try to balance for 30 seconds. Repeat two times, relaxing in between.
3. Switch to your right leg and repeat Steps 1–2 to complete one set.

Try to work up to holding your balance for two minutes. If you have difficulty balancing with no hands, try placing your fingertips or one fingertip on a hard surface until you are able to balance with no hands. Try and relax—it makes it easier.

You can make this exercise more difficult by closing your eyes while you balance. Removing vision from the picture requires more work from your muscles. Here are some other variations on the Stork:

- Once you have mastered standing still on one foot, try swinging your arms like you are running in place.

- When this is easy, hold water bottles or light weights in your hands and swing them.
- For even more challenge, fold up a bath towel so that it is several inches thick and do the Stork while standing on it. Be careful not to cheat by gripping the floor or the towel with your toes.
- If you are a golfer, mix in the Stork to balance your golf swing by taking your address position for a normal short iron shot and slowly lifting your back foot off the ground while maintaining your spine angle. Hold your foot 4 inches off the ground for 30 seconds and then lower it. Repeat this on your other foot.

Toe Raise

This exercise helps you coordinate the balance of your whole body as you shift your weight forward and stay aligned. It's not as easy as you might think to do this without wobbling.

1. Stand with your shoulders over your hips, hips over your knees, and knees over your ankles. In other words, line up.
2. Focus your eyes on a spot on the ground 25 degrees in front of you.
3. Lift your weight slowly off your heels and balls of your feet so that you are balancing on your toes.
4. Return slowly and in a controlled way to a flat-footed position, being careful not to jerk from side to side.
5. Repeat nine times to complete one set.

If you need some support during this exercise, stand behind a chair and use your fingertips to balance yourself.

Hip Flexor

This is another way to dynamically engage your balance, now on one leg in the forward plane. It requires core strength as well as your eyes, inner ear, and brain.

1. Stand next to a sturdy surface, such as a chair. If you need to use your fingertips for balance, do so.
2. Raise your right leg slowly off the floor like you are marching, then lower it. Engage your core, and do not bend forward at the waist. Repeat 10 to 15 times.
3. Switch to your left leg and repeat 10 to 15 times to complete one set.

Make this exercise more difficult by removing your fingertips from the chair (if you are using it) and even more difficult by closing your eyes.

Side Leg Raise

We move in all planes of motion daily. This exercise trains your balance in lateral motion.

1. Stand next to a sturdy surface, such as a chair. If you need to use your fingertips for balance, do so.
2. Raise your right leg to the side and hold it 6–12 inches off the floor (as shown in Photo 72), then lower it. Engage your core and do not bend forward at the waist. Repeat 10 to 15 times.
3. Switch to your left leg and repeat 10 to 15 times to complete one set.

Make this more difficult by removing your fingertips from the chair (if you are using it) and even more difficult by closing your eyes.

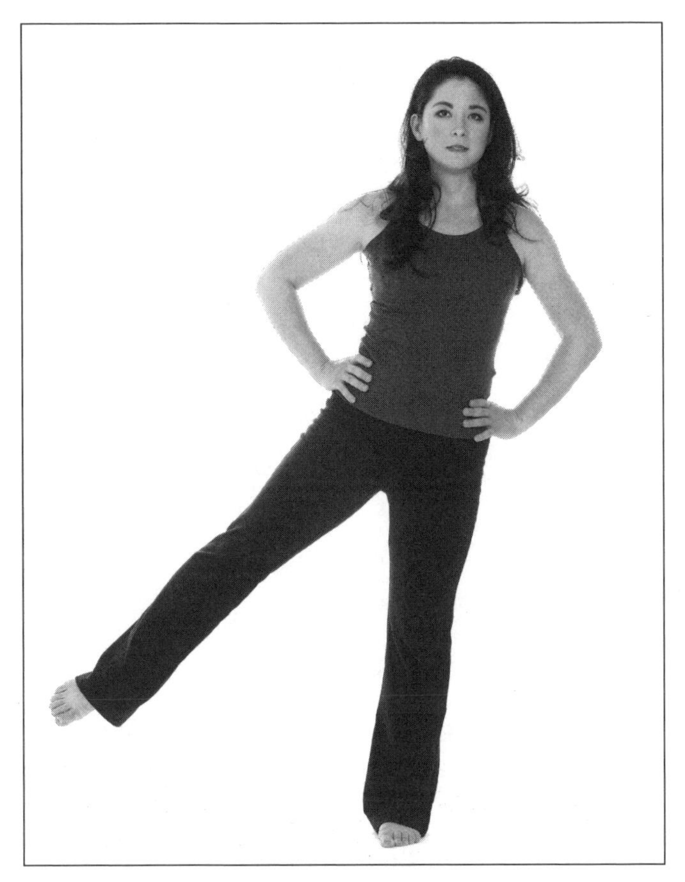

Photo 72

Walk the Line

This exercise can be difficult, even when sober, especially with your eyes closed.

1. Choose a straight line in front of you, such as a tile floor, and walk along it, with one foot directly in front of the other.
2. Walk backward to the starting point, still along the straight line.

Try this exercise first with your arms extended out to the side for balance, and then with your arms at your sides. When this is easy, do it with your eyes closed.

EXTRA FOR EXPERTS

You probably think the balance exercises described here sound simple, and you are right. They are simple, yet many people are surprised by how wobbly they are when they try them. Once you have the simple balance exercises under control, you can progress to more dynamic balance challenges using a BOSU ball (which looks like half a beach ball on a round plate). Performing any of the balance exercises described above gets harder when you engage your whole body while standing on a BOSU ball.

Here are some extra balance exercises for experts.

Chop Progression

Even though this exercise is performed standing on two feet, you do it holding a medicine ball or dumbbell. The movement of the medicine ball or weight in several planes of motion forces your body, eyes, and brain to engage together to keep you upright.

1. Stand with your legs shoulder-width apart and hold a medicine ball or dumbbell over your head.
2. Lower the ball or weight down between your knees in a squatting motion, keeping your back straight.
3. Stand and raise the ball or weight back up over your head. Repeat the sequence 10 to 15 times.
4. Take the ball or weight from high right to low left and back again. Repeat the sequence 10 to 15 times.
5. Take the ball or weight from high left to low right and back again. Repeat the sequence 10 to 15 times.

To make this exercise even harder, perform it while standing on a BOSU ball. If you are really expert, close your eyes.

CONE TOUCH

Ready for the hard stuff? This dynamic equilibrium exercise puts you on one foot while in motion. For best balance, engage your core and focus your eyes.

1. Place an object about waist high one yard in front of you.
2. Stand on one leg and reach for and touch the object while maintaining your balance.
3. Repeat this 10 to 15 times, then switch legs.

To make this exercise harder, lower the height of the object in front of you or stand on a BOSU ball.

You can do these balance exercises between parts of your resistance work (the "C" part of F.A.C.E.—carrying a load). If you do, you get two of the F.A.C.E. components of fitness in during the same time period. In other words, instead of just doing resistance (rest, resistance, rest) or balance (rest, balance, rest) in two separate time periods, you do both (resistance, balance, resistance, balance). You can do this because the balance exercises are not strenuous and probably don't require rest in between.

Equilibrium and balance are easy to ignore until you need them, and then it is way too late. Because the last thing anyone needs is to fall down, it pays to take the time to test your balance and use a few of the balance boosters given here every day.

WHAT YOU'VE GAINED SO FAR

Now you have covered the four components of fitness after 40 and are ready to F.A.C.E. your future in a smart way. It seems like a lot, but it will seem less overwhelming once you work the exercises into your muscle memory (yes, your muscles have memory and your mind will remember how it feels to do the exercises), know your target heart rate range, and know how much weight you should be carrying.

I hope what you have gained is not simply a list of exercises to perform but a real understanding of why you are going to do them. I will help you put it all together in Chapter 10 and you will then have a plan for fitness after 40.

HOME**WORK**

Before moving on, if you haven't already done so, take a minute to perform the balance test that appeared in this chapter. How old is your balance? If you felt wobbly during the test, seize the moment and perform one of the balance exercises described above, and practice it until you have memorized the exercise and can perform it without peeking at the book. Then memorize another balance exercise. Keep adding to your repertoire daily. Then, the next time you find yourself with a free minute (while pumping gas or waiting in line at a store, perhaps), you can invest in your equilibrium and balance.

NOTE

1. Wright, Vonda J., and Brett C. Perricelli, "Age-Related Rates of Decline in Performance Among Elite Senior Athletes," *American Journal of Sports Medicine* 36(3): 443–450 (2008).

"There is a difference between interest and commitment. When you're interested in doing something, you do it only when circumstances permit. When you're committed to something, you accept no excuses, only results."

—Art Turock, motivational speaker and author of *Getting Physical*

CHAPTER **TEN**

10

The Six-Week Jump Start to Mobility Plan—Your 20 Minutes to Burn

"I'm just so busy, I don't have *time*!"

Time is the most common excuse my patients give me for not taking control of the 70 percent of their health and aging that are governed by daily lifestyle decisions. The fact is that if we don't take time to invest in our health now, we will be forced in the future to take time to care for the diseases of sedentary living! You've heard me say it before and I'll say it again: 70 percent of your health and aging is controlled by the lifestyle and mobility choices *you make today!*

Only *20 minutes* of mobility each day can decrease your chance of early death by 20 percent and dramatically decrease disease in your future! Everybody has "20 minutes to burn"!

In the first edition of *Fitness After 40*, I gave you an amazing library of exercises to F.A.C.E. your future, and I taught you how to design your own fitness program. These step-by-step exercises (plus 24 new ones, added especially for this edition) are all featured in Chapters 6 to 9 of this second edition. What I've learned, however, since the first book was published is that many of you want a very specific plan to jump-start your mobility. I kept hearing: "Just tell me what to do and I'll do it." And I get that!

In this chapter, I give you my nine 20 Minutes to Burn exercise bricks and teach you how to combine them into a 20-, 40-, or 60-minute total body routine. This way, no matter how much time you have, you can burn through a workout. In addition, I've rolled the 20 Minutes to Burn bricks into a six-week total body mobility plan to jump-start the best years of your life. At the beginning, in weeks 0–3, I gradually bring you up to speed with my approach to total body workouts via the four components of F.A.C.E.-ing your future. During weeks 4–6, your body and brain will come to love the jump start on mobility you are burning through.

Just a note: Do not be weary of my talk about "burning." Remember, no matter what your age or skill level, there is *never* a time when your body will not respond to the positive energy you pour into it! I have tested my approach with hundreds of people after they have turned 40, 50, 60, and beyond, and they have loved it. Human beings are designed to move, and I guarantee you—regardless of whether you are a veteran masters athlete or you have not stepped away from the couch in 20 years—my Six-Week Jump Start to Mobility Plan and the 20 Minutes to Burn exercise bricks will not only change your body but will change your mind about what active aging can be.

INVESTING IN YOUR MOBILITY WITH A PLAN

The advice on the pages that follow is offered as a suggestion for getting you started. I hope you will use it as a template and think through what you have learned to customize a schedule that really works for you. When you invest your time in strategic planning, you own your regimen. And if you take ownership, you will be more likely to follow through.

If you stick with the plan, you will love the way your body feels at the end of six weeks. And if you continue to push, you will be amazed by what you will be able to do after 12 weeks. Seriously! Here are the basic steps you need to take before you either make your own plan or follow my jump start plan.

- *Ask yourself: "What do I want to do 12 weeks from now?* Set a distance, choose a race, or otherwise decide what you want to do. Think about your future.
- *See your doctor and get permission to start exercising.* Answer the health assessment questions in Chapter 7.
- *Make exercising nonnegotiable.* Plan around your exercise time. Don't just fit it in if you can—because you won't.

- *Set up a way to be accountable*. Tell all your family, coworkers, even strangers what you are going to do. Write it in your calendar, set an alarm in your PDA, put it up as your screen saver.
- *Establish a reward*. Feeling great is going to be an amazing reward, but perhaps you should buy yourself a special treat. Better yet, plan to race in some vacation spot.
- *Use my Six-Week Jump Start to Mobility Plan or write your own plan based on my example*. Do this today. Why wait? See the week-by-week plan in Table 2 later in this chapter. Remember to include:
  - F—Flexibility: daily
  - A—Aerobic exercise: three to five times, moderately, per week
  - C—Carry a load: three times per week (use the 20 Minutes to Burn exercise bricks)
  - E—Equilibrium/balance: daily

You are going to love my 20 Minutes to Burn exercise bricks as much as the hundreds of runners I've taught them to have. They are fun, fast-paced, and make a great workout. Plus, they get results *fast*.

INTRODUCING THE 20 MINUTES TO BURN EXERCISE BRICKS

Each of the following nine 20 Minutes to Burn exercise bricks gives you a "hot" and intense total body workout. Depending upon your needs, these bricks can be modified to serve either as the "A" (aerobic exercise) or "C" (carry a load) component of your commitment to F.A.C.E. your future. It will become abundantly clear how this all fits together once you read more about the Six-Week Jump Start to Mobility Plan.

Each brick, which comprises five individual exercises, should be performed in a 20-minute circuit. In other words, with good form, you should burn through each individual exercise for 45 seconds and then recover for 15 seconds before beginning the next exercise. (Note: This may not necessarily correspond to a complete "set" as defined in the earlier chapters. That's perfectly okay. The most important thing is to keep your heart rate up and maintain good form.) One five-exercise circuit should take you five minutes. Perform the circuit four times for a total of 20 minutes.

Now I want you to peek ahead and take a look at Table 2. Do you see the entries for Cardio Burn, Lunch Burn, Plyo I Burn, and so forth? These entries show how each of the Burn bricks can be utilized in the Six-Week Jump Start to Mobility Plan. You can either follow the plan in Table 2 that I designed and perform the brick assigned for each particular day, or—if you are designing your own workout—you can choose any one of the nine basic Burn bricks on the days you are committing to "A" or "C" activities, and blast your way to best health.

Do you have more time? Great! Then "sizzle" by stacking two 20 Minutes to Burn hot aerobic workout circuits. You can either choose from the nine basic circuits I designed, or you can mix and match individual exercises to create your own circuits. Or maybe you *really* want to burn. Fantastic! Spend 60 minutes and get a "burn" you won't forget by stacking three 20 Minutes to Burn bricks together.

The detailed, step-by-step instructions for each of the exercises in this chapter appear in Chapter 8. When you're first getting started with your new routine, you might need to refer back to that chapter from time to time if you haven't yet memorized each exercise. But after you've done a particular Burn circuit a few times, your muscle memory will kick in and you'll probably find that you won't need to consult previous passages.

I designed the following pages to serve as "cheat sheets"—providing quick visual references of each of the exercises in the circuit. In the spirit of the Fitness to Go philosophy, you can photocopy the page you need for a particular day (or even take a picture of it on your phone!) and literally tuck the circuit in your pocket. What can be easier than that? No excuses, now. Let's get started!

Cardio Burn

This Burn circuit is slightly different from the others in that you engage in one activity for the entire 20 minutes. What varies during that time is the level of intensity with which you perform the activity. (Remember the *fartlek* approach that we've discussed? Here is where you can put that philosophy into practice.)

Here's how you do a Cardio Burn. First, pick an activity. It might be jumping rope, climbing stairs, running (either in a park or on a treadmill), rowing, biking, swimming—you name it. Now, engage in that activity following this sequence:

1. Perform five minutes of slow warm-up.
2. Do two minutes of "fast burn." In other words, quickly get up to your MaxHR and maintain it throughout this period.
3. Take three minutes of slow recovery.
4. Repeat Steps 2–3 three times for a total of 20 minutes of Cardio Burn.

Lunch Burn

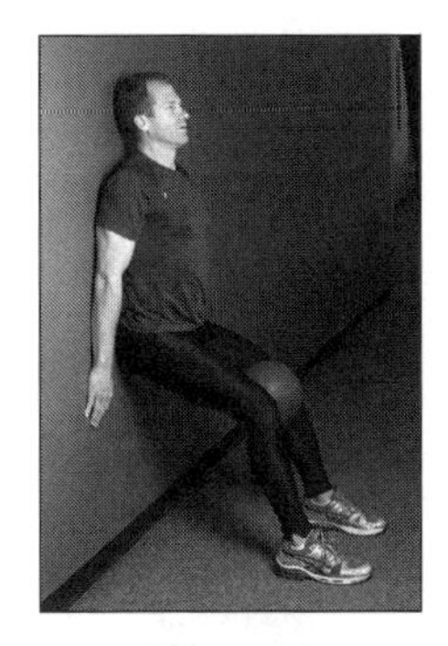

Photo 55

Short Arc Wall Squat
(See page 172)

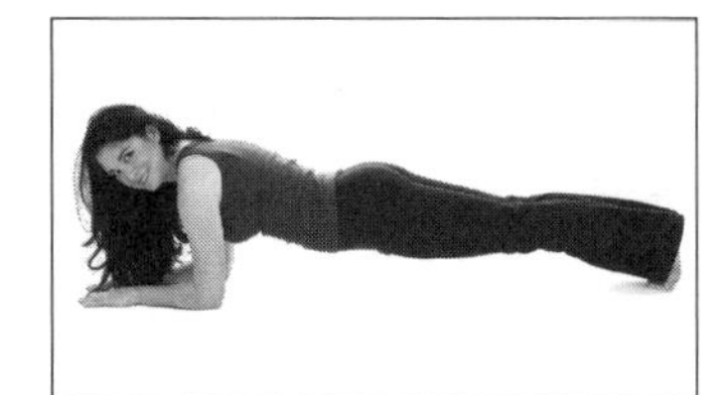

Photo 42

Plank
(See pages 161–162)

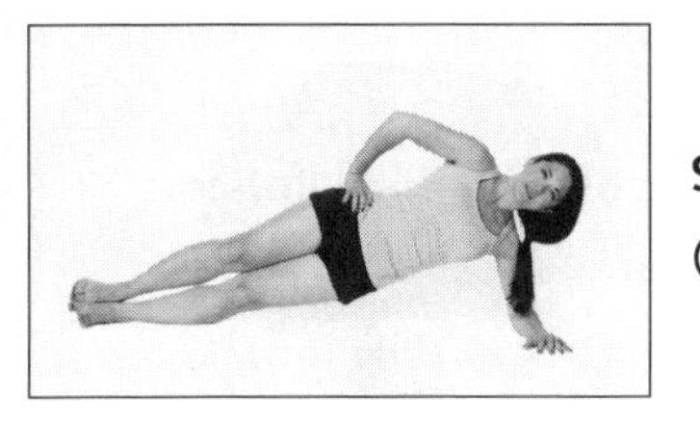

Photo 43

Side Plank
(See pages 162–163)

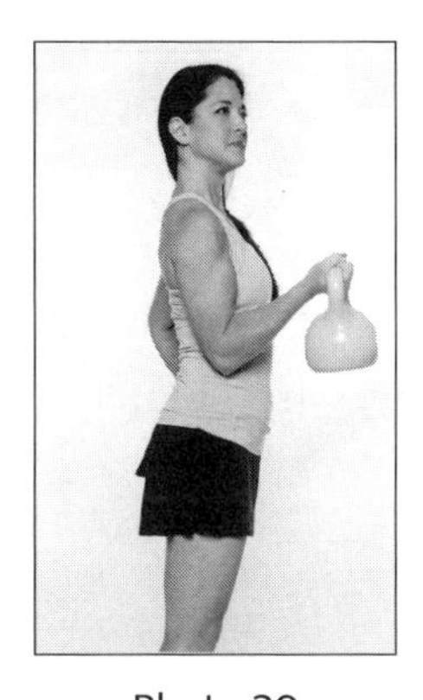

Photo 39

Biceps Curl
(See page 158)

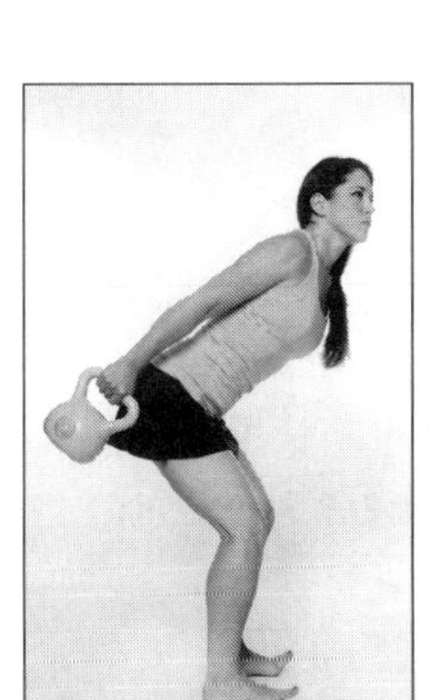

Photo 40

Triceps Extension
(See page 159)

Arm Burn

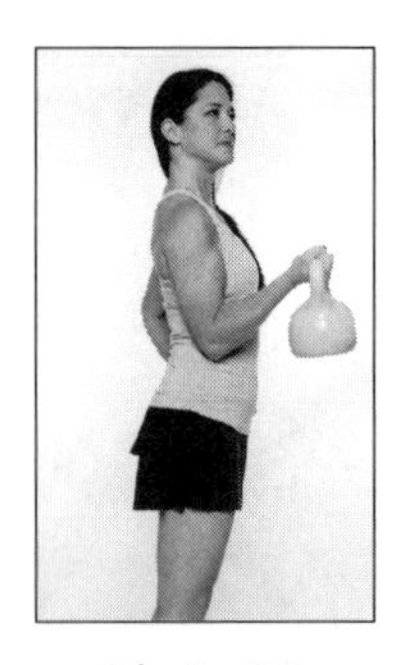
Photo 39

Biceps Curl
(See page 158)

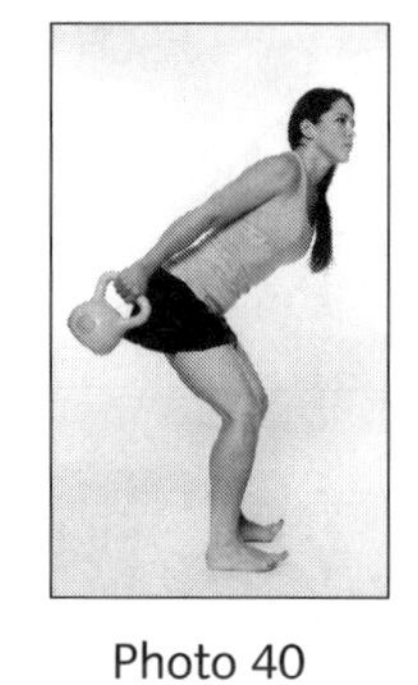
Photo 40

Triceps Extension
(See page 159)

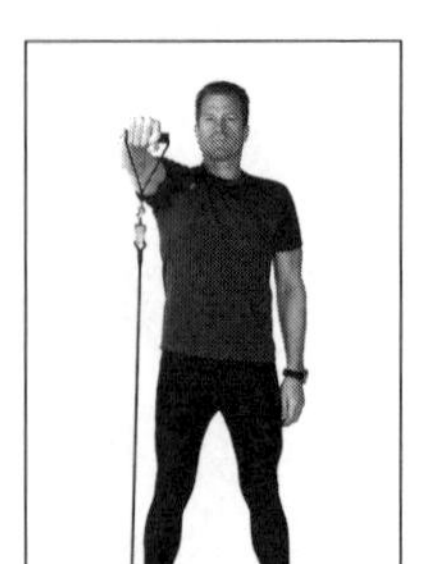
Photo 32

Forward Rotator Cuff Raises
(See pages 154–155)

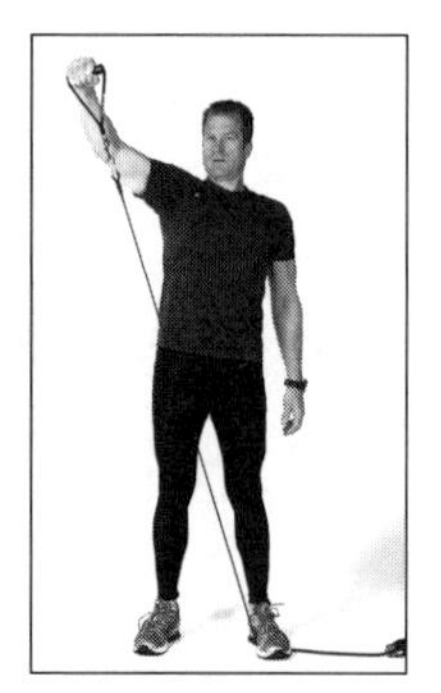
Photo 33

Across-the-Body Rotator Cuff Raises
(See pages 154–155)

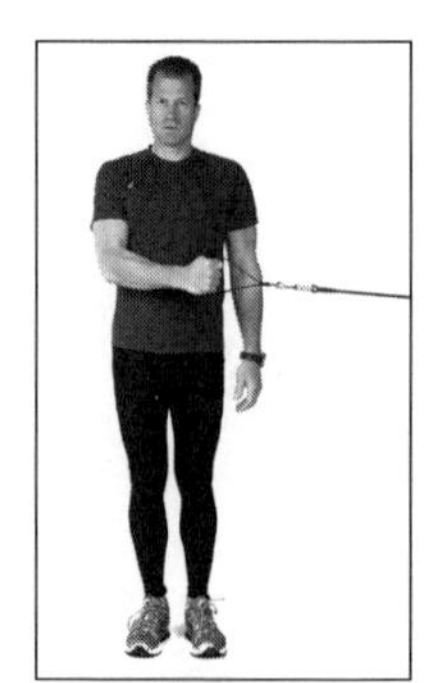
Photo 34

External and Internal Rotation
(See pages 155–156)

Leg Burn

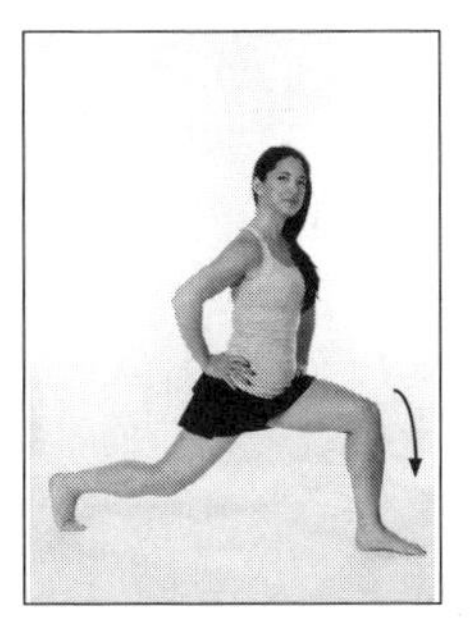

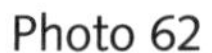

Photo 62

Runner's Lunge

(See page 179)

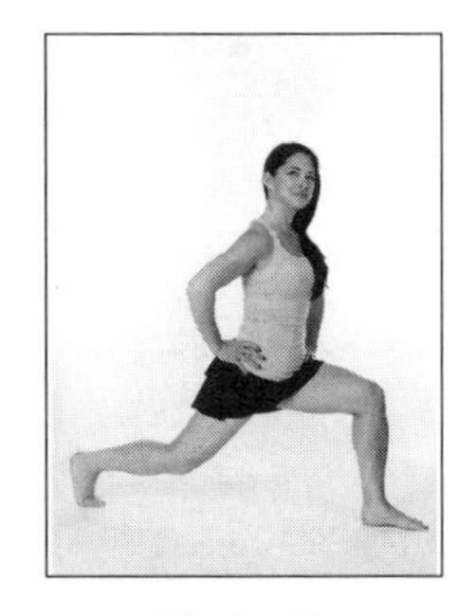

Photo 62

Reverse Split Squat

(See page 180)

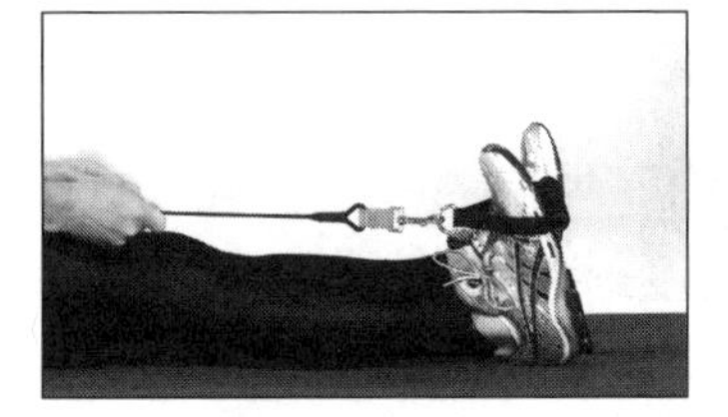

Photo 63

Plantar Flexion/ Dorsiflexion

(See pages 180–182)

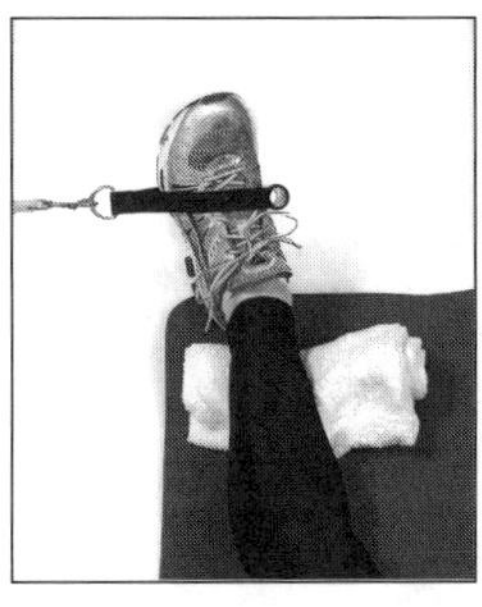

Photo 67

Ankle Inversion

(See pages 182–183)

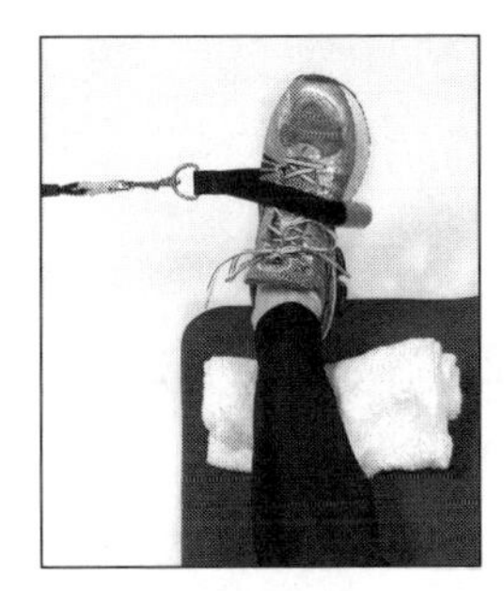

Photo 68

Ankle Eversion

(See pages 182–183)

Butt Burn

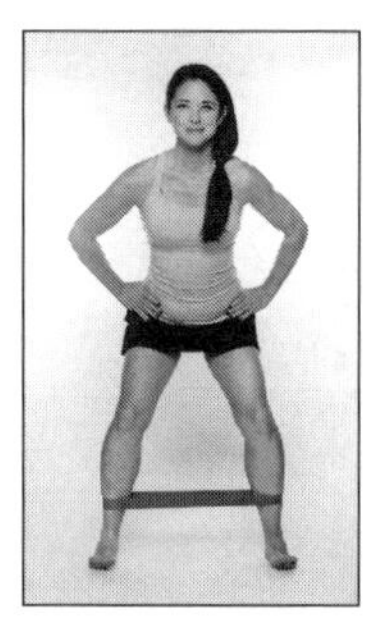

Photo 60

Monster Walk
(See page 177)

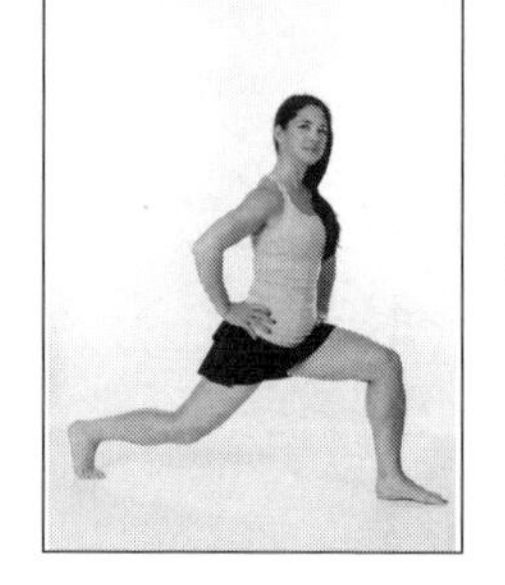

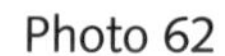

Photo 62

Runner's Lunge
(See page 179)

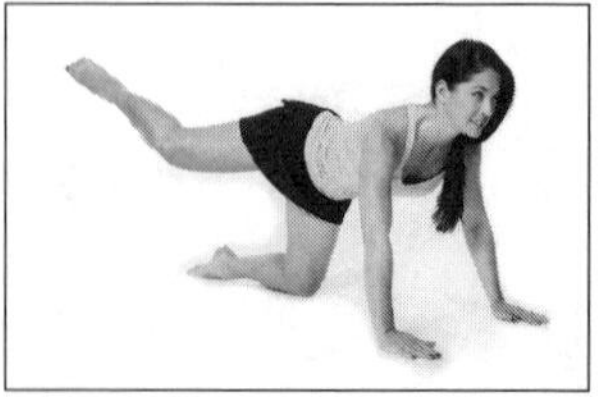

Photo 61

Fire Hydrant
(See page 178)

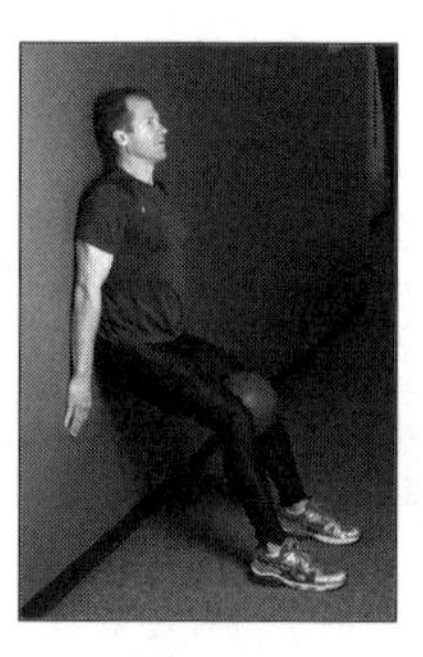

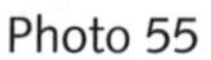

Photo 55

Short Arc Wall Squat
(See page 172)

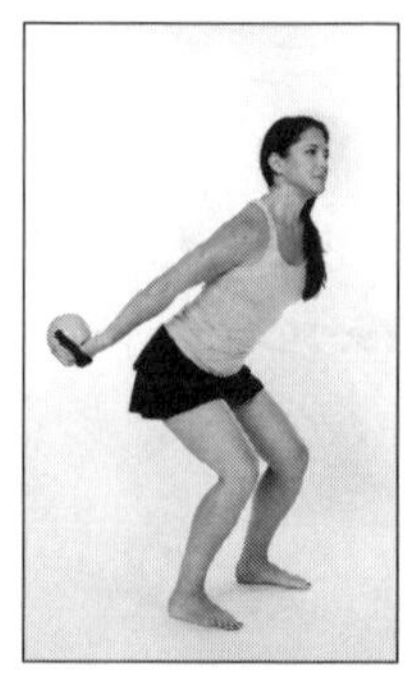

Photo 69

Vertical Jump
(See pages 185–187)

Core I Burn

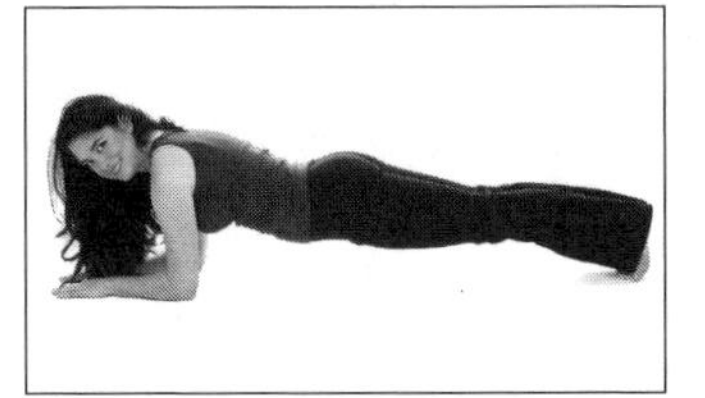

Photo 42

Plank
(See pages 161–162)

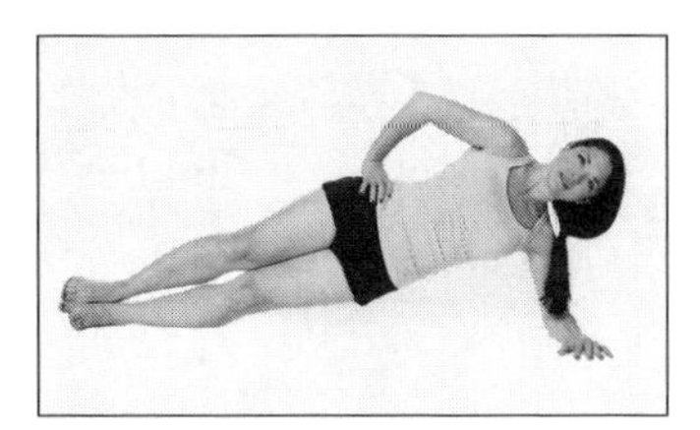

Photo 43

Side Plank
(See pages 162–163)

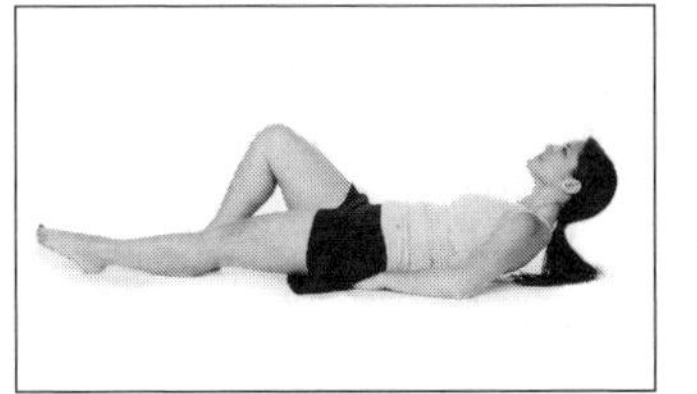

Photo 46

Classic Crunch
(See page 166)

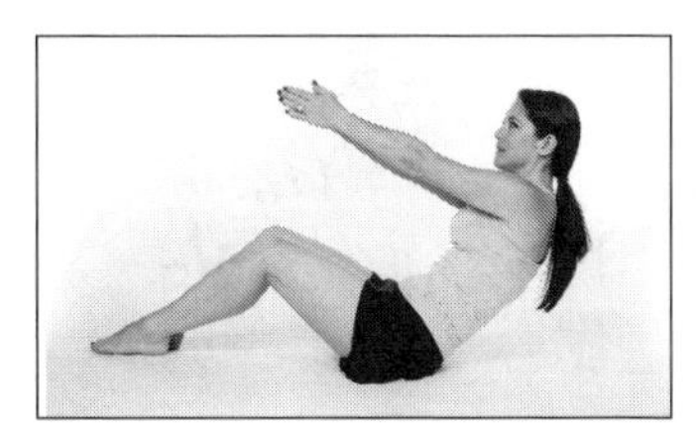

Photo 47

Russian Twist
(See pages 166–167)

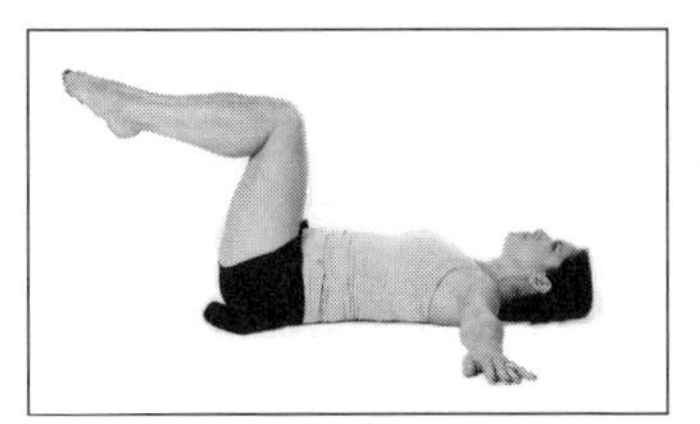

Photo 49

Oblique Twist
(See pages 168–169)

Core II Burn

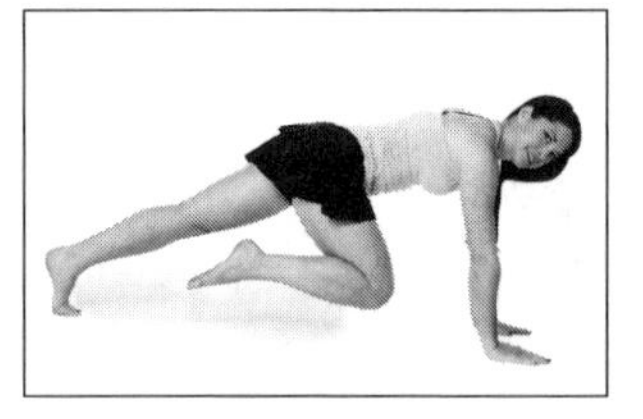

Mountain Climber
(See pages 169–170)

Photo 52

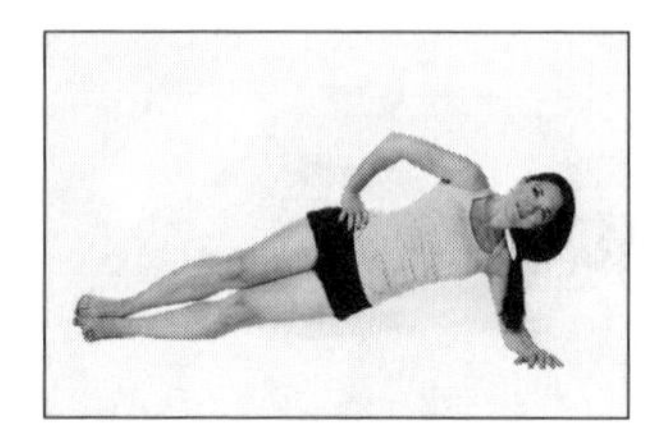

Side Plank with Upper Leg Swing
(See pages 163–164)

Photo 43

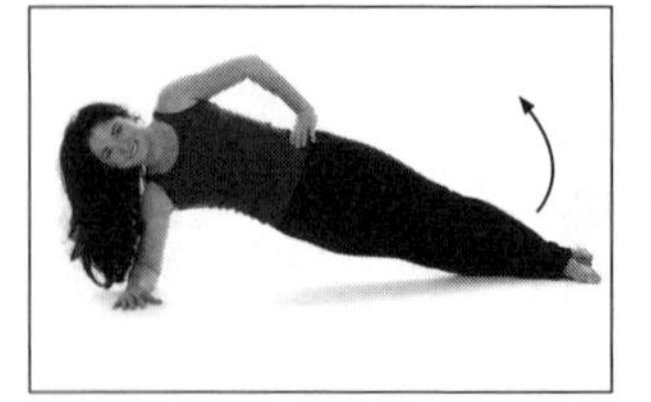

Side Plank with Upper Leg Lift
(See pages 164–165)

Photo 44

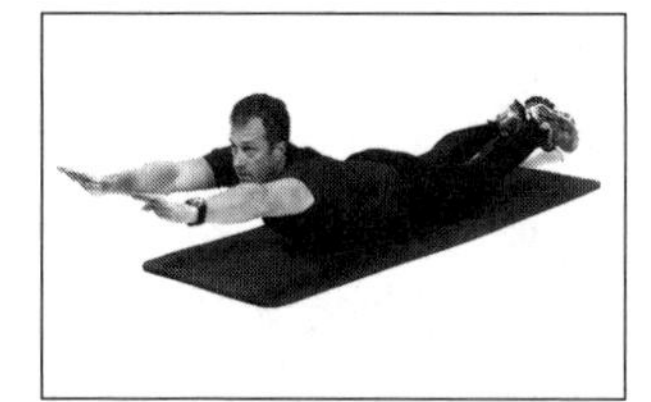

Superman (and Woman!)
(See page 165)

Photo 45

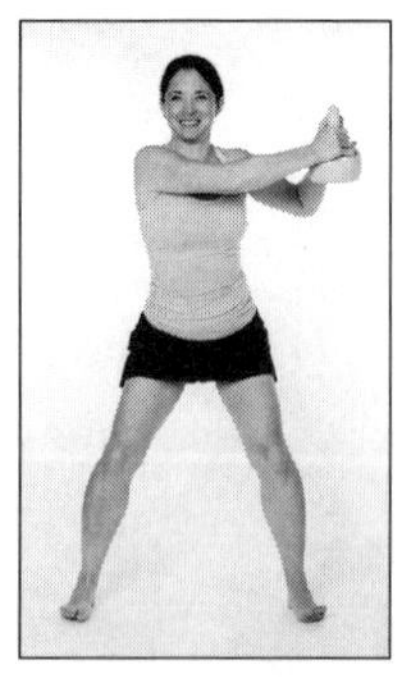

Kettle Bell Twist
(See pages 170–171)

Photo 53

Plyo I Burn

Side Shuffle
(See page 187)

Monster Walk
(See page 177)

Grapevine Step
(See page 188)

Standing Broad Jump
(See pages 188–189)

Forward Jump and Stick Landing
(See page 189)

Pylo II Burn

Two-Way Hop (Right and Left)
(See pages 189–190)

Two-Way Hop (Front and Back)
(See page 190)

Triple Jump
(See pages 190–191)

Power Skip
(See page 191)

Lateral Hop with Balance
(See pages 191–192)

INTRODUCING THE SIX-WEEK JUMP START TO MOBILITY PLAN

Most of my patients find that the Six-Week Jump Start to Mobility Plan is an amazing way to get moving toward their best life. Of course, you're welcome to modify it to suit your individual needs and schedule. Refer to Table 2 as you read through the following week-by-week descriptions.

Week 0

Start on a weekend or when you have more time. Test your shoes. Always warm up for five to 10 minutes prior to exercising. (For suggestions, see the discussions on Foam Rolling and Dynamic Stretching and Warm-Up in Chapter 6.) My plan starts you out with a simple brisk walk on Saturday and introduces you to your first 20 Minutes to Burn brick on Sunday.

Week 1

This week, you are going to continue your new aerobic habit on three days. You can use the 20 Minutes to Burn bricks as your "A" (aerobic exercise) if you burn with an intensity that gets your heart rate up. Otherwise, the Burn bricks should be used to "C" (carry a load), which you will start in week 2.

In the example in Table 2, "A" is done on Tuesday, Thursday, and Saturday during week 1, but you can choose any three days you wish. Notice that *Lunch Burn* appears on Tuesday of week 1; this presumes that you'll do it intensely and get your heart rate up (so it qualifies as an "A"). On the second aerobic day of the week, add "F" (flexibility) *after* you exercise. Static stretch only warm muscles.

Table 2. The Six-Week Jump Start to Mobility Plan

Week 0

	Goals	Monday	Tuesday	Wednesday	Thursday	Friday	Saturday	Sunday
A	Add 2x						30 min. brisk walk	20 min. *Cardio Burn*

Week 1

	Goals	Monday	Tuesday	Wednesday	Thursday	Friday	Saturday	Sunday
F	Add 2x				X		X	
A	Increase to 3x		20 min. *Lunch Burn*		30 min. brisk walk		20 min. *Cardio Burn*	

Week 2

	Goals	Monday	Tuesday	Wednesday	Thursday	Friday	Saturday	Sunday
F	Increase to 7x	X	X	X	X	X	X	X
A	Continue 3x	30 min. brisk walk or 20 min. *Cardio Burn*		30 min. brisk walk or 20 min. *Cardio Burn*		30 min. brisk walk or 20 min. *Cardio Burn*		
C	Add 3x		20 min. *Arm Burn*		20 min. *Leg Burn*		20 min. *Core I Burn*	

Week 3

	Goals	Monday	Tuesday	Wednesday	Thursday	Friday	Saturday	Sunday
F	Continue 7x	X	X	X	X	X	X	X
A	Continue 3x	30 min. brisk walk or 20 min. *Cardio Burn*		30 min. brisk walk or 20 min. *Cardio Burn*		30 min. brisk walk or 20 min. *Cardio Burn*		
C	Continue 3x		20 min. *Lunch Burn*		20 min. *Butt Burn*		20 min. *Core II Burn*	
E	Add 7x	X	X	X	X	X	X	X

Week 4

	Goals	Monday	Tuesday	Wednesday	Thursday	Friday	Saturday	Sunday
F	Continue 7x	X	X	X	X	X	X	X
A	Increase to 4x and stack bricks	30 min. brisk walk or 20 min. *Cardio Burn*		30 min. brisk walk or 20 min. *Cardio Burn*		30 min. brisk walk or 20 min. *Cardio Burn*	30 min. brisk walk or 20 min. *Cardio Burn*	
C	Continue 3x		20 min. *Arm Burn*		20 min. *Leg Burn*		20 min. *Core I Burn*	
E	Add 7x	X	X	X	X	X	X	X

Week 5

	Goals	Monday	Tuesday	Wednesday	Thursday	Friday	Saturday	Sunday
F	Continue 7x	X	X	X	X	X	X	X
A	Continue 4x and stack bricks	20–30 min. walk, run, or *Cardio Burn*		20–30 min. walk, run, or *Cardio Burn*		20–30 min. walk, run, or *Cardio Burn*	20–30 min. walk, run, or *Cardio Burn*	
C	Increase to 5x and stack bricks		*Core II Burn & Lunch Burn*		*Arm Burn & Leg Burn*		*Butt Burn*	
E	Cont. 7x	X	X	X	X	X	X	X

Week 6

	Goals	Monday	Tuesday	Wednesday	Thursday	Friday	Saturday	Sunday
F	Continue 7x	X	X	X	X	X	X	X
A	Continue 4x and stack bricks	20–30 min. walk, run, or *Cardio Burn*		20–30 min. walk, run, or *Cardio Burn*		20–30 min. walk, run, or *Cardio Burn*	20–30 min. walk, run, or *Cardio Burn*	
C	Increase to 5x and stack bricks		*Arm Burn & Leg Burn*		*Core I Burn & Butt Burn*		*Plyo I Burn*	
E	Cont. 7x	X	X	X	X	X	X	X

Key: F = Flexibility (Chapter 6), A = Aerobic Exercise (Chapter 7), C = Carry a Load (Chapter 8), E = Equilibrium/Balance (Chapter 9)

Week 2

This week, you are going to focus on "C" (carry a load). Three days is enough. When selecting Burn bricks for your weekly plan, it is best to challenge alternating body parts. In other words, do a lower extremity aerobic workout one day followed by an upper body aerobic workout the next day (e.g., *Arm Burn* on Tuesday and *Leg Burn* on Thursday).

Note: In my example weeks, you will notice that "A" activities fall on Monday, Wednesday, and Friday and that "C" activities fall on Tuesday, Thursday, and Saturday. (The "F" component is now daily and should immediately follow your "A" or "C" workout.) However, this is the time when you can deviate from my plan and start to stack the 20 Minutes to Burn bricks, if you so choose. Personally, I find it easier to do "A" and "C" both on the same day, with "F" at the end.

Week 3

You are now F.A.C.E.-ing your future by adding the "E" (equilibrium/balance) exercises, either throughout the day or as part of your concentrated workout. Like flexibility exercises, equilibrium exercises are best done every day. Continue the "A" (aerobic) and "C" (carry a load) components of your workout as before. If you are not able to fit it all in according to the plan, do your best. Doing something is better than doing nothing. Remember: Accentuate the positive. No defeatist self-talk. In week 3, if you do FAE on Monday, then Tuesday is FCE.

Weeks 4–6

Continue your F.A.C.E. regimen into week 4. It seems like a lot, but if you move steadily through your workout without a lot of standing around in between the different parts, you can fit it all in in about an hour. For instance, you might spend 10 minutes with a dynamic warm-up, 20 minutes on aerobic exercise, 20 minutes on carrying a load, and 10 minutes stretching and cooling down. Then, each of the last two weeks, either increase your "A" (aerobic exercise) time by at least 10 percent or add a day (three to five days is the goal).

Remember, as we spoke about in Chapter 7, make a specific, strategic plan for each day of the week that includes date, time, location, activity, intensity, and duration/distance. For instance, using the sample plan in Table 2, the plan for Monday of week 3 might be:

> Monday (FAE) 5:30 P.M.: North Park Circle—10-minute dynamic warm-up; 20-minute jog with MaxHR around 70 percent; 10-minute static stretch. Note to self: Take gym bag to the office and work out on the way home.

It may be rocky at first, as the movements, equipment, and training in general are unfamiliar, and you may consider hanging it all up. Don't do it. Feeling awkward is very normal, but soon you will develop a routine or a rhythm to your workouts and you will flow from one component to the next.

I like to do my aerobic and resistance work all on the same day. I warm up, run or spin on a cycle, get a quick drink, and then immediately go to carrying a load with my arms and legs. Then I stretch . . . *and feel so good.*

REAPING THE REWARDS

By the end of six weeks, you will feel really different from the way you did when you started—I promise. Your body will feel stronger, your mind will be more confident, and you may even begin to look forward to the adrenaline rush that is a part of aerobic exercise. Changing your life does not happen overnight. It is a strategic commitment. Your body will change after a month or six weeks of working, so stay focused and don't lose heart.

If the six-week plan charted in Table 2 works for you, use it. My goal, however, is that you will *own* your future by planning strategically for it. *Make your own plan*. Copy Table 3 from the end of this chapter, fill it in, and hang it on the refrigerator door.

As you finish a daily workout and feel some part of it went especially right or especially wrong, make a note of it. Not only is it fun to look back over the road you have traveled but the information can help you with your next plan.

At the end of six weeks, evaluate how you are doing:

- How do you feel while exercising?
- Do you need to rearrange your schedule to make it work for you?
- Do you have any injuries?
- Are there any barriers, mental or physical, that you need to work through?

When you have evaluated your first six weeks, make a second six-week plan to reach the 12-week goal that you set for yourself earlier in this chapter, when you were making your plan. As we discussed in Chapter 7, in order to improve, you need to overload your body and make it work harder. In your second six-week plan, covering weeks 6–12, you need to increase the frequency, intensity, or time (duration) of your workouts to move to the next level.

To ramp up in the second six weeks, you might graduate from walking to running (if that is your goal) or try *fartlek* training, which can be as simple as alternating walking and running. (First you start with a five-minute walk, followed by a five-minute run. Continue alternating walking and running for a minimum total of 20 minutes.) Over the next several weeks, decrease the time you walk and increase the time you run until you can run for 20 to 30 minutes without stopping. Once you can do that, you can simply ramp up your workouts by increasing your running times. You can also increase your intensity by keeping the total amount of time the same but running at a faster pace. If your goal is a sport other than running, you can also ramp up your workouts by increasing the frequency, distance, or intensity.

It is so exciting for me to think about you doing this because I know it is life-changing stuff. It makes me so happy to hear my patients tell me, in excited voices, the stories of their progress. I see the confidence in their faces and the swagger in their walk. You can do this. *Onward!*

Table 3. My Six-Week Plan for Getting off the Couch and onto My Future

	Monday	Tuesday	Wednesday	Thursday	Friday	Saturday	Sunday	Goal
Week 0								
Week 1								
Week 2								
Week 3								
Week 4								
Week 5								
Week 6								

Key: F = Flexibility (Chapter 6), A = Aerobic Exercise (Chapter 7), C = Carry a Load (Chapter 8), E = Equilibrium/Balance (Chapter 9)

HOMEWORK

I'm serious when I say that everyone has 20 minutes to burn during the day. Take a few minutes right now and identify three times during the course of a typical day when you could invest 20 minutes in your best health. Might it be at lunch? Immediately after work? After dinner during the evening news? Every minute you move counts toward your fitness after 40. Start right now by choosing which burn workout you will start with, make a specific plan, and then *go!*

"The modern definition of fitness is not just aerobic capacity or muscle tone. True fitness needs to be from the foundation up and that means fitness for all the cells and tissues that make up your musculoskeletal frame."

—Nicholas DiNubile, M.D.,
author of *FrameWork*

CHAPTER **ELEVEN**

11

Maximizing Performance and Minimizing Injury

"I had been trying to do the same kind of workouts that I did in high school, and I was constantly getting strains and pains. I spent 50 percent of my time healing from my workouts."

I have heard variations of this statement from many of my patients. Either they do the same kinds of workouts they have always done, or they cram all their exercising into the weekend. These "weekend warriors" try to make exercise-cramming work for them because their weeks are crazy . . . activities, errands, and no scheduled time for exercise. When the weekend comes, they are free and they hit the gym or road or court with bravado. They ignore the fact that such a dramatic shift from inactivity to activity makes them prone to injury. Come Monday morning, these warriors are speed-dialing my office for an appointment. This was especially true during the Olympics and World Cup. People were so inspired that they flew out their doors to exercise. Many ended up in my office because you cannot regain your youth in a few days.

Sports injuries are way up for baby boomers. According to the Consumer Product Safety Commission, there was a 33 percent increase in the number of sports injuries in mature athletes between 1991 and 1998. A 1996–2007 epidemiologic study of Central European adults found injury rates doubled in masters-aged athletes.[1] And musculoskeletal injuries are the Number 2 reason adults and kids visit the doctor (the common cold is Number 1). In the Consumer Product Safety Commission findings, the highest number of injuries occurred while people were biking, playing basketball, playing baseball, and running, with the most common injuries in the ankle/leg, knee, shoulder, and lower back. Acute and overuse injuries are the primary reasons people stop exercising and the major causes of performance declines in masters athletes. The more we push the athletic envelope—whether we are longtime competitors or the sudden athlete leaping off the couch for the first time in years—injuries are always lurking in the wings, ready to sideline us if we don't learn to avoid them.

PRECAUTIONS YOU SHOULD TAKE WHEN BEGINNING TO EXERCISE

To optimize your fitness after 40, you need to harness not just the strength of your body but the wisdom of your age. This will help you make the best decisions when you begin to exercise.

- *Don't be a "weekend warrior."* Packing a week's worth of activity into a day or two is a recipe for disaster. Try to maintain a moderate level of activity throughout the week.
- *Learn to do your sport right.* Using proper form can reduce your risk of overuse injuries, such as tendinitis and stress fractures.
- *Remember safety gear.* Depending on the sport, this may mean knee or wrist pads or a helmet.
- *Increase your exercise level gradually.* Don't be a victim of the Terrible Toos (too much, too soon, too often, and with too little rest). The best way to progress without getting injured is to increase your workouts gradually.
- *Strive for a total body workout.* Incorporate cardiovascular, strength training, flexibility, and equilibrium exercises into your routine.
- *Engage in cross-training.* Mixing up activities like running, swimming, cycling, and rowing reduces injury while promoting total fitness.

INJURIES IN MASTERS ATHLETES

In 2005, the University of Pittsburgh conducted a survey of more than 2,500 Senior Olympians at the National Summer Senior

Games.[2] A majority of the athletes—89 percent—had experienced at least one sports-related injury since turning 50, and more than 50 percent had experienced up to five injuries. These injuries did not occur just because of a bad landing or acute incident. In fact, the majority of injuries in senior athletes are the result of overuse: workouts that are too frequent, too repetitive, and too intense. During the 2005 Senior Olympics, more than 60 percent of the injuries were attributed to overuse. Such problems commonly occur at the insertions of tendons and bone. In addition, 23 percent of the injuries were the result of falls. The athletes who reported having arthritis were twice as likely to have more than five injuries as athletes without the disease. They were also three times more likely to report knee injuries.

For aging athletes and adult-onset exercisers, the main problems reported are acute muscle strains and chronic tendinitis. The junction between the tendon and the muscle is especially vulnerable since the structure of the muscle is less "stretchy" in this area than in the middle of the muscle. In addition, when muscles are fatigued, they lose their ability to absorb energy and are less coordinated. This makes them susceptible to injury during so-called eccentric movement. ("Eccentric" means that the muscle is contracting as it is lengthening. This predisposes it to injury.)

Too much, too soon, too often, and with too little rest—these Terrible Toos predispose us to overuse injuries. Unfortunately, these problems are common in older athletes and often result from a condition called tendonosis. While tendinitis is the acute inflammation of the tendon, tendonosis is the longer term, cumulative effect of repetitive microtrauma to the tendon that does not properly heal.

The Achilles tendon, patellar tendon, rotator cuff tendons, medial epicondylitis (inside elbow), lateral epicondylitis (tennis elbow), and wrist tendons are all more vulnerable with aging. As we've discussed, as we age, our cells and tissues have less regenerative capacity than they did when we were younger. This leads to less durability of our muscles and tendons. Our musculoskeletal tissues also have a lower healing capacity, so it takes longer to recover between intense workouts. When not rehabilitated correctly, these overuse injuries can linger on and on, resulting in literally years of lost activity. This simply points to the fact I have been making throughout this book: As we age, we must not only become or remain active but be smarter about how we do it and F.A.C.E. our physical futures.

I experienced this myself as I aged. When I turned 30 and was only running, I developed a number of persistent injuries. I could almost predict that when I reached a certain level of training, I would pull my medial calf muscle or get hip pain. The muscle pulls often set me back a couple of weeks, which can devastate a race-training schedule. At age 40, I ramped up my training while also working on flexibility, lifting weights, and doing cross-training. I did not get hurt at all and managed to cut almost two minutes from my mile time.

You may have also experienced the pop, tear, and pain that sidelines you and leaves you wondering how in the world it happened or what to do next.

HOW YOU HEAL

From the moment a ligament, muscle, or tendon tears, your body goes to work to repair the damage. Here's what happens at each stage of the healing process:

- *At the moment of injury:* Chemicals are released from damaged cells, triggering a process called inflammation. Blood vessels at the injury site become dilated. Blood flow increases to carry nutrients to the site of the tissue damage.

- *Within hours of injury:* White blood cells (leukocytes) travel down the bloodstream to the injury site, either inside your body or on your skin, where they begin to tear down and remove damaged tissue, allowing other specialized cells to start developing scar tissue. Scar tissue is not the perfect way for us to heal; however, it is the way we do it. Only the bones are capable of regenerating without scars. All other soft tissues heal well but with scar tissue.
- *Within days of injury:* Scar tissue begins to form. The amount of scarring may be proportional to the amount of swelling, inflammation, or bleeding within. In the next few weeks, the damaged area will regain a great deal of strength as scar tissue continues to mature.
- *Within a month of injury:* Scar tissue may start to shrink, bringing damaged, torn, or separated tissues back together. However, it may be several months or more before the injury is completely healed.

WHAT DO WE DO WHEN WE GET INJURED?

Treating injuries begins before you get injured. Overtraining and overuse are the most common reasons for getting injured. Your muscles get tired during workouts and become inflamed and may feel sore. Your muscles and the tendons that hold them to the bone need time between intense workouts to recover adequately. By ignoring the ache, you are predisposing the formation of scar tissue from the persistent inflammation caused by too frequent workouts. Scarred tissue is more fragile than healthy tissue.

Here are the four rules to follow in injury prevention:

1. *Rule Number 1* is to exercise intensely every *other* day to give your body time to recover. As you've heard me say, make it work, then let it rest.
2. *Rule Number 2* is to mix up your workout to use different muscle groups. In other words, cross-train. In my chapters on aerobic exercise and critical strength, I always employ exercises that work more than one set of muscles and never use a weight machine. I want you to get a total body workout using different muscle groups during each circuit.
3. *Rule Number 3* is to warm up before exercising. This is as easy as using the Dynamic Stretching and Warm-Up in Chapter 6, walking for 10 minutes before you run, or setting the resistance on the stair stepper on low before you ramp up your workout. (Remember that the warm-up is not Static Stretching; these are separate activities. Also recall that you should not stretch prior to warming up.) You are simply trying to raise your core body temperature. Warm muscles and tendons are less brittle than cold muscles. The flexibility and foam rolling exercises in Chapter 6 are also a good way to prevent injury. While you do not want to stretch when cold, the stretches you perform daily will keep your body limber and prevent the formation of scar tissue during the exercise recovery period. The proper order for initiating a workout is to warm up, stretch, and then turn up the intensity.

As I mentioned, the most common injuries I see in senior athletes are to the leg and ankle, knee, shoulder, and lower back. Treating these injuries is preventing these injuries. The way we do this is called *pre-hab*. Pre-hab is simply strengthening the most injury-prone muscle groups before they ever get injured. Many of the exercises in the Fitness to Go sections in Chapter 8 are designed to pre-hab these four muscle groups. The stronger our muscles are, the less likely they will succumb to injury; therefore, strengthening our weak areas is key.

4. *Rule Number 4* for injury prevention, therefore, is pre-hab!

TREATING MINOR INJURIES WITH R.I.C.E.

Each letter of this acronym stands for one component of treating minor injuries.

- ***R = Rest***. After you hurt yourself, back off the intensity of your workouts and give your injured part a rest. This does not mean sitting around on a couch. Rest is an active process and may involve changing activities; you can cycle, swim, or walk instead of running. It may also require taking a day or so off. While you are resting, make sure you keep moving your injured joint and continue gently stretching your injured muscles. This will minimize scar tissue and stiffness while you heal.
- ***I = Ice***. Ice is so good for injury—what would we do without it? Place a bag of ice or an ice pack over your injured part and leave it there for 20 minutes several times a day during your recovery period, especially in the first 72 hours. An easy way to do this is to put the ice in a thin plastic bag (the kind from the grocery store work well) and strap it on with clear plastic wrap. Note that this is not the time for heat. Use heat only after the first 72 hours to warm up the injured body part prior to motion.
- ***C = Compression***. This is just what it sounds like. Compression does wonders for preventing and reducing swelling. Keep a cou-

ple of Ace elastic bandages around the house for just this purpose. When you get injured, gently wrap the bandage around the joint, starting farthest away from your heart and wrapping toward your heart. This helps your body absorb the fluid causing the swelling and move it back into your circulation instead of getting pooled (accumulated) at the injury site. This also helps you recover faster since your body must eventually reabsorb all the fluid it dumps at the injury site.

- ***E = Elevate***. Coupled with compression, raising an injured part as high as you can above your heart prevents and reduces swelling. When hurt, we temporarily lose our ability to control fluid at the injury site and so must help our bodies. If we don't elevate, fluid pools at the injury site, making healing more difficult.

So what if Rules Number 1–4 in treating injuries with R.I.C.E. didn't heal your injury or relieve your pain? Now what? Stop playing or exercising immediately. Ice the injured area as soon as you can, and elevate the body part above your heart. These measures will help minimize the amount of swelling and inflammation that occurs and will decrease the pain. Taking an NSAID (nonsteroidal anti-inflammatory drug) such as ibuprofen or naproxen will also decrease inflammation and pain. Ice and elevation are key in the first 72 hours after injury.

Next, you should temporarily back off your activity level. This does not mean that you sit on the couch! Getting back in the game is an active process. However, if you are unable to bear weight on the limb you hurt or can't move the joint, you should see your doctor.

Even if your injury is minor, your body still tries to protect itself by getting stiff. Gently move the joint through its full range of motion, fully straight and fully bent. Do this several times a day. Gentle stretching aids in the healing of a pulled muscle with less scar tissue. While you are recovering from your injury, you also can still maintain your fitness by working the other body parts that remain well. For instance, if you hurt your shoulder, use a stationary bike; if you hurt your leg, lift weights with your arms or swim with a buoy between your legs.

When I rehabilitate one of my surgery patients, I follow a specific rehab order for returning her to sport. This order is the same for getting you back into the game. Regain your full range of motion first. When this is back, you may begin strengthening the muscle you pulled or the muscles around the joint you injured. At the same time, you should focus on training your injured joint to balance again. We lose our ability to balance well when we are injured. This is especially true for our knees and ankles.

ACUTE AND CHRONIC INJURIES

Acute injuries, such as sprained ankles, strained backs, or fractured hands, occur suddenly during activity. Signs of acute injury include:

- Sudden, severe pain
- Swelling
- Inability to place weight on a lower limb
- Extreme tenderness in an upper limb
- Inability to move a joint through its full range of motion
- Extreme limb weakness
- Visible dislocation or break of the bone

Chronic injuries, such as anterior knee pain, stress reactions, or iliotibial band pain, usually result from overusing one area of the body while playing a sport or exercising over a long period. These injuries creep up on you and you may not be able to pinpoint the exact time they began. Signs of chronic injury include:

- Pain that increases when performing an activity
- A dull ache when at rest
- Swelling and redness

SPORT-SPECIFIC SETBACKS

Each sport uses a different set of muscles, and overuse can result in sport-specific injury patterns. To avoid these setbacks you need to identify vulnerable areas and work to preemptively strengthen them.

Running

Most running injuries result from too much road pounding. Remember the Terrible Toos discussed earlier in this chapter (too much, too soon, too often, and with too little rest)? Runners are especially susceptible to them. Another reason why runners tend to get injured is that most only run. They don't do anything to strengthen their cores or buttocks, let alone stretch their hamstrings or other leg muscles.

The most common running injuries are bursitis over the hip bone (ITB syndrome), anterior knee pain, Achilles tendinitis, shin splints, and plantar fasciitis (sharp heel pain when you first get out of bed in the morning). What you need to remember is that we are a kinetic chain from our toes to our backs; in other words, everything is connected and works together. This means that even something simple can have a widespread effect. For example, having a stiff big toe that will not flex when you roll through a stride can force your weight to the outside of your foot, which changes the forces across your knee while you bend it by pulling your kneecap to the outside. This increased patellar force can put too much pressure on the kneecap cartilage or on the patellar tendon below the kneecap and cause them to become irritated. The pain is worse when your quadriceps are not strong enough to keep your kneecap on straight. Tight hamstrings can cause you to have a shorter stride or walk with bent knees. This forces your hips to bend more and may cause lower back pain. We really are all connected.

So what does a runner have to do to stay injury-free? Start with your big toe. Flex it up and down and move it all around in a circle. To land correctly, you need 70 degrees of flexibility in the big toe. Next, make sure your calves, hamstrings, and quads are well stretched. Our muscles are most efficient and most supple at their optimum length. Next, even runners need to work on keeping their legs, hips, and cores strong. Use the "Fitness to Go: Your Butt, Quads, and Knees" section in Chapter 8 as a start. For one simple exercise for your lower body, try the Prisoner Squat.

Finally, don't forget your most important piece of equipment for runners: the shoes. When your shoes are too old, they no longer support your efforts. Even if the upper cloth part of your shoes still looks good, realize that the soles last only 350 to 500 miles before their engineering fails. It works well to have several pairs that you rotate through instead of completely wearing out a pair before having to break in another. Chapter 15 tells you how to think about purchasing shoes.

As discussed previously, tendinitis is the inflammation of overworked tendons. For AOEs who run (or who swim or cycle, for that matter), acute tendinitis from sudden increases in activity intensity can slowly progress to tendonosis. Tendonosis is chronic structural changes to the tendon, when the normally white, gleaming, pulled-taffy appearance of the tendon is changed to a gray, amorphous, painful lump. The best treatment for tendinitis and tendonosis is prevention. Don't just A.C.E. your future: You must F.A.C.E. it. In other words, flexibility is key.

Finally, AOEs can quickly develop muscle imbalances that lead to injury. Shin splints are one of the most common muscle imbalance injuries—you know, the aching down the front of your legs that hurts with each step. Refer to the "Fitness to Go: Your Lower Legs" section in Chapter 8 and look at the leg exercises you can do to avoid shin splints. If you do get them, treat them initially with an ice massage, active rest, and NSAIDs. To perform an ice massage, freeze water in a paper cup. Then tear back the cup edges to expose about an inch of ice, which can then be rubbed over the front of your legs.

Since the original edition of *Fitness After 40*, I have developed a large library of videos specifically targeted to keep runners "on the road and out of the doctor's office." Please take advantage of the amazing video tips and exercise circuit videos found at www.drvondawright.com/media/.

SUDDEN RUNNER'S SYNDROME

Those of you just starting out or those who are weekend warriors who "start out" every weekend are especially prone to a sudden onset of new leg pain, which takes the form of muscle soreness and tendinitis. Your muscles and tendons are probably wondering what they ever did to you to deserve such pounding. They scream back by getting all hot, bothered, and sore.

As adults, most of us develop delayed muscle soreness from sudden increases in exercise intensity two days after the workout day. The first day after, you feel a little muscle burn, but the real hobbling soreness comes 48 hours later. Muscle soreness is caused by the accumulation of multiple microtears in your muscle fibers during exercise. These tears form in proportion to the amount and type of exercise you are doing. Eccentric muscle contractions—those contractions that force the muscle to lengthen as it is firing—cause the most microtears. Examples of eccentric contractions include running downhill (or down stairs) and lowering weights. Soreness also occurs due to the buildup of lactic acid. Lactic acid, which is the by-product of anaerobic (without oxygen) metabolism, builds up in our muscles under intense conditions.

Muscle soreness generally fades away in a few days. In the meantime, you should recover actively. Drink a lot of water immediately after exercise, and cool down actively to wash the lactic acid out of your muscles (for instance, walk after you run to cool down). Instead of exercising intensely the next day (which I never recommend), take a walk or do a low-impact workout, making sure to gently stretch after you warm up, or get a massage. Not only does massage feel good but it can reduce some of the swelling that causes the muscle pain. Ice and NSAIDs can also take the edge off the muscle soreness and inflammation. As your soreness fades, warm up well and resume your exercise.

Swimming

While swimming is an excellent way to stay in shape and avoid the pounding of the road, aging shoulders are very susceptible to rotator cuff injury. The rotator cuff lives in a house of bone. That is, the main rotator cuff tendon, the supraspinatus (above the spine of the shoulder blade), travels under a ceiling of bone called the acromium (the bone you feel when you place your fingers on the top of your shoulder) and over a floor of bone called the humeral head (the top of your upper arm bone). Between these two bones is a small space through which your main rotator cuff muscle lives as it goes away from the neck and ends on the outside of your humerus. When you swim, the repetitive stroke action of your arms impinges or pinches the tendon between these two bones and causes tendinitis or even tearing. This is worse if the shoulder girdle is weak. This tendon is slow to heal because it has a poor blood supply.

Keep your rotator cuff strong with the exercises in the "Fitness to Go: Your Shoulders and Arms" section in Chapter 8, and avoid using hand paddles, which increase the upward pressure of the humeral head on the supraspinatus muscle.

Cycling

Cyclists get injured not only because of the Terrible Toos but also because equipment is so important to the overall kinetics of the ride. Here are a few things to keep in mind about your bike and riding in general:

- For a road bike, keep your frame size 2.5 cm (about 1 inch) from crotch to top-tube. For an off-road bike, keep it 7–15 cm (about 3–6 inches).

- Seat height should allow approximately 30 degrees of knee bend at the lowest point. A low seat forces the knee to bend more and may cause knee pain.
- The forward tip of the saddle to the center of the handlebars should equal the distance from the tip of your elbow to your long finger. Although a longer crank length gives you a mechanical advantage, it also forces your hips and knees through a larger range of motion and increases your risk of injury.
- If you are still using toe clips, exchange them for bike shoes to keep the ball of your foot over the pedal axel. This also helps to avoid foot nerve compression injuries and numb toes.

An important way to avoid cycling injuries is to get your bike fitted to your body at a reputable bike shop. In this process, they take a variety of measurements, only one of which is the distance between your feet and your seat, and adjust each component of your bike so that it is more efficient for your body.

To avoid the other cycling pitfalls that cause knee injury, modify your training to restrict intensity when you are sore or injured, keep your cadence (pedal speed) greater than 90, and limit hill workouts until your symptoms subside. Keep your quads, hamstrings, and calves flexible. If you have access to a therapist with electrical stimulation, you can use it to strengthen both types of muscle fibers (fast- and slow-twitch) and equalize your medial and lateral quad strength (usually, the medial or inside portion of the quads is weaker than the lateral or outside portions). Orthotics or wedges may compensate for foot pronation (flat feet). You should also refrain from doing squats and lunges while you are injured.

Cyclists may develop Achilles tendinitis from the repetitive dorsifflexion (ankle flexed up) during the power phase of cycling or if the seat is too low. If your foot does not flex up enough or is flat, you are at a higher risk for plantar fasciitis (inflammation of the tight tissue on the bottom of your foot). Forefoot pain can be avoided by preventing excessive resistance (too much pressure) in a low cadence (slow pedal speed).

CAN I EXERCISE WHEN I'M SICK?

Moderate exercisers are known to spend about 50 percent fewer days sick than non-exercisers, but what should we do when we do get sick? Drink lots of fluid, get some rest, and eat chicken soup—just like your mother said.

- If you have a cold with a stuffy nose, cough, aches, and pains, you can get back on track with intense exercise when your symptoms resolve and you can breathe.
- Walking is good for you any time and will not make your cold worse.
- If you have severe flu, a fever, or severe fatigue, you should give yourself one to two weeks to recover and then start exercising slowly.

ARTHRITIS: OH, MY ACHING JOINTS

Stiffness, aching, grinding, swelling, outright pain—these are all symptoms of arthritis and can be a barrier to staying mobile as we age. The good news is that there are many ways to treat arthritis and get you back into the game.

The Arthritis Foundation reports that 50 million people in the United States have arthritis. What exactly is this common affliction associated with aging? Simply, it is the wear and tear of the cartilage that lines the end of your bones. Normally, cartilage is smooth, glistening, and white, and two cartilage-covered bones moving across one another in our joints are virtually frictionless. In fact, they are smoother than ice. When the cartilage begins to wear down, though, like potholes in a road, the surface loses its smooth finish. This is when the stiffness and aching set in.

ThermaCare asked baby boomers about living with arthritis. Sixty-seven percent reported having weekly muscle or joint pain. Of those with pain, 69 percent said they simply worked through the pain to remain active; 90 percent believed their pain was treatable and were looking for new and better ways to treat it.

If you have arthritis, this is a marvelous time to have it. What I mean by this is that there is virtually a smorgasbord of treatments to try while remaining active. Some of them are discussed below.

Arthritis Home Remedies

Most people with arthritis experience a gradual onset of aches and pains in their joints and don't immediately make their way to a doctor's office. Here are some home therapies to try:

- ***Heat therapy***. Warmth feels great on stiff joints in the morning when you wake up, before exercise, or while you are sitting in one place for a long time (like at work) and are creaky when you get up. The easiest way to apply heat is with one of the several available arthritis heat wraps. These disposable wraps warm up to 104°F, are air-activated, and last between eight and 12 hours. The warmth increases the blood supply to the joint and helps you move it through a range of motion. I like ThermaCare HeatWraps since they conform to the joint and last 12 hours. You can also use a heating pad, a moist towel warmed in the microwave (be careful not to burn yourself), or a hot water bottle. I do not recommend the variety of arthritis creams and gels that make the skin feel warm. Generally, they do not change the temperature of the actual soft tissues surrounding the joints, plus they leave you smelling medicated.

- ***Ice therapy***. Ice is an excellent remedy after activity, at the end of a long day, after exercise, or any time a joint feels painful. Not only does this simple solution calm the inflammatory process going on in your knees but it confuses the pain pathways and decreases pain. A minimum of 20 minutes is necessary. Apply the ice pack or simply a bag filled with ice and wrapped in a thin towel over your joint. (Our skin gets thinner with age, and the towel prevents damage.) Generally, you should use ice after activity and reserve heat for warming up and getting going in the morning.

- ***NSAIDs***. Most of you will say that you are not "pill people," but this class of drugs does not simply mask the pain—it actually treats the source. Nonsteroidal anti-inflammatory drugs (e.g., ibuprofen, naproxen, etodolac, celecoxib) are a class of medications that work directly at the cellular level to halt inflammation. In arthritis, you experience pain because of the toxins released from the inflammation of an arthritic joint. One purpose of this body reaction to injury is to clear away the cellular debris that happens with injury. The substances made by the body are powerful; I often describe what is going on in an inflamed joint as "chemical warfare." These toxins then inflame the tissue surrounding them, and a circular pattern of pain and inflammation arises. You must nip the cycle in the bud and get rid of the toxins.

I would not suggest taking NSAIDs if they really did not make a huge impact on your discomfort. Taking them for arthritis is not like taking an aspirin when you have a headache. NSAIDs are most effective if taken regularly over a course of days. They are usually taken several times a day, and it takes several days to build up a therapeutic level in your blood. NSAIDs can have some side effects. They can increase your blood pressure or upset your stomach. Ask your doctor if taking NSAIDs is all right for you. This is especially important if you have stomach problems.

- ***F.A.C.E. regimen***. You thought F.A.C.E.-ing your future was related only to how to exercise, didn't you? Every patient who comes to my office with arthritis pain is put on a flexibility, exercise, resistance, and balance program. I usually begin by sending them for six weeks to physical therapy to jump-start their program, and then they transition to a fitness program if they are not already on one.

Keeping your joints supple by stretching is important since arthritis tends to make joints even stiffer than what would occur in one's body due to the effects of aging alone. Aerobic exercise is key for maintaining overall musculoskeletal health. With arthritis, you may need to modify what you do to keep active. For instance, swim in a warm pool, cycle, or spin to take the load off your leg joints; use the elliptical machine instead of running. The fitness component is also important in maintaining a healthy body weight. Excess weight is felt by your joints! Did you know that your knees bear five to seven times your body weight with every step? This means that for every extra 10 pounds you weigh, your knees feel like they are carrying 70 extra pounds. Stated positively, if you can lose the extra 10 pounds you are carrying around, your knees effectively lose 70 pounds!

• If you have arthritis, it is vital that the muscles surrounding your joints become and remain strong in order to absorb some of the impact of daily activity. The key to your knees being able to handle this stress is the strength of your quadriceps. As every one of my patients can recite for you, "The quads are the key to the knees!" These four giant muscles on the front of your thighs can significantly assist your knees in bearing the load of your body if they are strong and decrease the pounding and pain your joints feel.

• ***Balance and fall prevention***. You must retrain your muscles and muscle/brain pathways to maintain balance. As discussed in Chapter 9, as we age, we lose our ability to balance well, and arthritis makes this worse. Not only does our balance decrease in one knee with arthritis but it also decreases in the opposite knee. We don't know exactly why this occurs; we simply know that it does and adds up to a double whammy.

• ***Active rest***. Finally, if you have pounded out an intense workout and your joints are sore, rest them. This does not mean sitting on the couch for several days. Instead, get on a bike and spin, row, use the elliptical, or work out your upper body alone one day. Rest is great . . . when it is active.

In our survey of 2005 Senior Olympians, there was a definite association between having arthritis and injury. People with arthritis were twice as likely to have five musculoskeletal injuries and three times more likely to have injuries around the knees. This is because of quadriceps weakness and altered balance. The physical therapy prescription for my patients with arthritis therefore reads:

- Heat/cold therapy
- Joint range of motion

- Strengthening of quadriceps, core, and hips
- A fitness program that transitions to a home program
- Balance and equilibrium training

Arthritis Remedies from Your Doctor

While you are capable of eliminating much of your arthritis pain with the home remedies I've suggested, sometimes they are simply not enough. Your doctor has several ways to help you with your arthritis pain.

- ***Joint injections***. Physicians use two categories of joint injections to relieve arthritis pain: steroid injections and joint lubrication. Steroid injections have been around for a long time and consist of injecting the joint with a mixture of numbing medicine, such as steroids and lidocaine or marcaine. The point of this injection is to decrease the pain and inflammation of arthritis. These injections usually last an average of three weeks, and most physicians give only three a year to any joint. I tend not to use steroids unless my patients have excruciating pain. I prefer to use joint lubrication with a class of injection called hyaluronic acid. (There are currently five of these on the market. Four are purified from the comb of roosters, and the fifth is grown in bacteria and then purified for injection.) The hyaluronic acid works to decrease inflammation and lubricate the joint. It causes the joint lining to secrete substances that feed the remaining cartilage. Hyaluronic acid injections work best in early arthritis and can be effective up to six months or longer. They are given once a week for three to five weeks and can be repeated every six months if patients receive significant relief.

Not long ago, I began the fourth round of hyaluronic acid injections into the left knee of one of my patients, Mark. A 54-year-old insurance salesman, he always hurries in between his business appointments for his knee injections. Mark lies down on the exam table and pulls up his trouser leg, I inject his knee, and he runs out the door to his next meeting. Not much inconvenience for the six months of pain relief and the increased function he gets.

When he was in high school, Mark had some kind of knee injury, and now his left knee has significant arthritis with narrowing of the joint space and bone spurs, called osteophytes, around the bone edges. This arthritis caused his knee to ache day and night and had begun to limit his activity. Worse yet, Mark began to gain weight from being more sedentary. Today, his right knee is completely normal, with wide-open joint spaces and no pain, but his left knee needs help. When he first came to me and I diagnosed where his pain was coming from, he was a little skeptical of my three-prong regimen of NSAIDs, physical fitness, and hyaluronic acid injections. After I made my case for why these three approaches are key, he agreed to try them. Well, two years later and starting his fourth round of twice-yearly injections, Mark is a true believer in this method. For Mark and many of my other patients, arthritis does not mean the end of their active lives. It simply means we have to harness all the treatments available to keep them going.

- ***Joint bracing***. Knee arthritis can cause legs, in particular, to move from straight to bowlegged or knock-kneed. This is because as one side of the knee wears down, the joint on that side collapses. Most people wear down the inside compartment of the knee first and end up with bowlegs. Braces can "unload" the affected side of the joint by pushing on the opposite side and effectively straightening the leg again. For instance, if you have arthritis on the inner side of your knee and develop bowlegs, the brace will unload that side by pushing against the outer side of the knee. The problem with knee braces is that they work only if they are worn daily, and many people simply put them in the closet.

Custom braces are made especially for you and must be ordered by your physician. The stretchy knee sleeves you can buy in the pharmacy are not effective in unloading the knee and are not what I am describing here. (Some of my patients like the sleeves, though, because they make them more aware of their knees and they feel more stable.) A study found that for decreasing knee pain and increasing stability, the custom braces were the best but the sleeves were better than nothing.

- ***Alternative/complementary therapies***. Many patients ask me if using herbs or alternative therapies will help their arthritis. Although many people swear by products such as chondroitin sulfate, glucosamine, and shark cartilage, there is currently no convincing evidence in the medical literature that these remedies are better than a sugar pill. A recent study, however, shows that acupuncture can relieve arthritis pain. To this end, I tell my patients that as long as the alternative therapy is not hurting them—and they think it is possibly helping—then they are welcome to take it.

- ***Arthroscopic joint debridement***. "Washing the joint out" by surgically removing loose tissue or debris in the joint using a small camera and instruments inserted through tiny incisions has not been found to be effective for long-term treatment of arthritis pain. The only true indication for arthroscopic surgery with arthritis is if the person has mechanical catching or locking (which feels like popping, snapping, or sharp pain) because of a torn meniscus or a loose body floating around in the joint. The meniscus is the wedge-like rubbery cushion located between the femur (thighbone) and tibia (shinbone) and is responsible for supporting 80 percent of the body's weight. It thus protects the ends of the bones from grinding on each other. The menisci (you have two in each knee) are among the most commonly injured parts of the knee. They are separate from the cartilage that coats the ends of the bones. If you want to think about the knee in layers going from the thighbone to the shinbone, each side would go: thighbone, cartilage, meniscus, cartilage, shinbone.

If you play a contact or noncontact sport, you may tear the meniscus by twisting the knee, pivoting, cutting, or decelerating. You can injure your meniscus without any trauma since the collagen weakens and wears thin over time, setting the stage for a degenerative tear. Arthroscopic surgery is useful if loose bodies (pieces of cartilage or bone that break off) are getting caught in the joint. The surgery eliminates the mechanical symptoms but does not touch the aching pain of arthritis. I always make this distinction clear to my patients.

My Arthritis Protocol

After I examine my patients and go over their X-rays with them, we discuss their arthritis and the treatments available. I initially treat them using the following four-pronged approach:

1. NSAIDs to decrease inflammation and pain
2. Physical therapy with a transition to a fitness program to work on range of motion, strength, balance, and weight control
3. Injections of hyaluronic acid to lubricate and feed the remaining cartilage
4. Creation of an anti-inflammatory environment in the body with the smart nutrition described in Chapter 13

Every athlete at some point experiences injury. As a mature athlete or adult-onset exerciser, injury and arthritis may be a part of your challenge to stay active. Your goal should be to prevent those repetitive injuries that sideline your future and listen to your body when it tells you it is hurting so you can treat it actively.

HOME**WORK**

It is important to identify your recurring injuries in order to work on the mechanical and strength problems that cause them. Take a minute now to list your most common injuries, and then another minute to reflect upon them:

- What are they?
- When do they happen? (It may be a particular time of year, for instance, or during a specific sport.)
- What are you doing when they occur? (A specific action may initiate the injury.)
- Are these injuries simply from ramping up volume or speed too quickly, or do you have pain that makes the other side compensate and get injured, too?

Keeping an accurate history of your injury patterns will help you prevent them by strengthening your weak body areas and understanding which activities leave you vulnerable.

NOTES

1. Kammerlander, Christian, M. Braito, Stephen Kates, Hans-Christian Jeske, Tobias Roth, et al., "The Epidemiology of Sports-Related Injuries in Older Adults: A Central European Epidemiologic

Study," *Aging—Clinical and Experimental Research* 24(5): 448–454 (2012).

2. Wroblewski, Andrew P., Francesca Amati, Mark A. Smiley, Bret Goodpaster, and Vonda Wright, "Chronic Exercise Preserves Lean Muscle Mass in Masters Athletes," *Physician and Sports Medicine* 39(3) (2011).

"We can rebuild him. We have the technology.
We can make him better than he was.
Better, stronger, faster."

—Oscar Goldman in the *Six Million Dollar Man*

CHAPTER TWELVE

12

Healing with Steel

When the pain and functional disability of arthritis are causing a daily decline in the quality of life of one of my patients, we discuss total joint replacement. Many people cringe when they hear those words. However, we are talking about replacing parts of your body that no longer serve you with parts that will. It may be a little hard to grasp when you first think about it, but we want to make you a little "bionic," like the Six Million Dollar Man.

Today, doctors are capable of replacing many joints in the body, from your knuckles to your ankles, but the knees and hips are the most commonly replaced joints. The American Academy of Orthopaedic Surgeons estimates that between now and the year 2030, there will be a 673 percent increase in the number of total knee replacements and a 174 percent increase in the number of total hip replacements performed. The increases will be the result of the aging of our population and improvements in joint technology.

I was taught and I teach my residents that "we don't treat X-rays, no matter what they look like; we treat patients." This means that we don't replace a joint just because a person's X-ray shows a lot of arthritis. We replace a joint only when a patient has a high grade of arthritis, has tried conservative measures, and says either "Doc, I can't take the pain another day," or "Doc, you have got to help me get my life back." Then we are ready to discuss joint replacement.

Orthopaedic surgeons suggest total joint replacement to treat pain, increase mobility, support functional independence and psychological well-being, and help people return to sport! Total joint replacement is no longer thought of as a procedure that buys time for a person's joint as he walks toward death but instead is viewed as a way to reclaim mobility. In other words, joint replacement is now associated with a longer life!

MY PARENTS' STORY

In June 2013, both of my parents had total joint replacements—on the same day! Neither of them could take the pain they were feeling any longer, but more importantly, both had to get back to a normal, mobile life. Like many of you, they had stopped doing the things they loved and were living a more sedentary existence. This resulted in weight gain and increased medical problems in a very short amount of time. Prior to surgery, my mom's mobility was so limited that she had rarely left the house for two years.

I asked one of my partners to replace my mom's knee and another to replace my dad's hip, and after three- and two-day hospital stays, respectively, they came home to begin renewed, mobile lives. Make no mistake: Rehabilitation from a total joint replacement is a huge commitment. They both worked hard to rebuild muscle and stamina, but the results have been truly life-changing!

My dad entered his first post-surgery race, the Liberty Mile, two months after his joint replacement and finished his "walk/run" in 15 minutes. It was a true victory of body, mind, and spirit. He continues to walk/run daily, and although I no longer allow him to tax his joint with long-distance running, he is living the life he loves and is back to training groups of beginning runners.

My mom has transformed into the athlete she never was. For my whole life, she moved through her day at a thousand miles an hour but never really worked out. Since her knee replacement, she now not only takes Zumba classes but she walks on the treadmill and swims in the pool, has minimized her medical problems, and has returned to being the fast-speed mom I've always known. At 74 years old, she had her first "sports"-related injury—a sprained ankle because she was moving too fast in Zumba class. Today, she is considering a "hip-hop aqua aerobics class." I love it!

Being healed with steel has transformed my parents' lives!

CONSIDERING JOINT REPLACEMENT

There are many issues to consider when deciding to undergo joint replacement. Traditionally, doctors waited until patients were as old as possible before replacing their joints because the average total joint lasts only between 10 and 15 years. At that point, many joints require revision surgery to replace worn parts.

For patients, waiting until some arbitrary old age to have a joint replaced means suffering with the pain and debilitation of arthritis, cutting back their activity, becoming sedentary, and in many instances needing to take chronic pain medications—all while waiting until the magic year when a surgeon finally decides they are old enough.

Today, there is a trend to replace worn-out joints earlier in order to give the person another 10 to 15 years of active life. Yes, this means that some people will require additional surgery for joint revision at some point, but it also means that instead of sitting around getting fat and debilitated, many people can resume or increase the activity in their lives. In addition, improved joint technology and new joint materials are making it possible for replacement joints to last longer, so revision surgery might not be necessary for more than 15 years.

I have a patient named Larry. He is a giant man towering more than 6′5″ and once weighing almost 500 pounds. Larry had been an athlete in high school and college, and after graduating, he kept consuming the calories of a high-level athlete even though he stopped exercising like one. The weight eventually added up. Larry remained as active as he could and coached his son's football team until he just couldn't take the pain in his knees anymore. His weight and natural anatomy had destroyed the cartilage in his knees, and he was walking around with bones grinding on bones like a mortar and pestle. At only 36 years old, Larry was no longer able to play with his five children and was beginning to have difficulty holding down his job.

Traveling from doctor to doctor, looking for an answer to his debilitating knee pain, Larry was told repeatedly that he was too overweight and too young for knee replacements. He was determined to get his life back, however, and over the course of a year lost nearly 200 pounds. However, his knees were still not participating in his life and were still causing him pain. When he finally came to see me, he was still young and a giant, but he had done the hard work of losing almost half his body weight. He was frustrated and almost in tears as I, too, expressed to him my concern about replacing his knees because of his young age.

As a surgeon, I had a decision to make. Did I sentence this young man to 15 more years of pain, disability, and a certain sedentary lifestyle by saying no to replacing his knees, or did I bite the bullet and give this man a license for mobility by replacing his arthritic knees with new ones made of cobalt-chrome? Both Larry and I knew he would certainly require revision surgery sometime in the future. But because my goal is to keep people as mobile as possible for as long as possible and prevent the ravages of Sedentary Death Syndrome, I replaced his right knee.

Larry flew through the three months of rehab without a hitch, and even at his first post-op visit, he came in beaming from ear to ear. The only pain left in his right knee was the incision pain. The grinding pain that had taken away his active life was gone. Over the course of the next year, Larry returned to work, began coaching his son's team again, and loved his new lease on mobility. He had such a life-changing experience with his first replacement that I replaced his left knee the same year. New knees gave life back to this young man so that he can again enjoy his children, wife, and job. He has continued to thrive over the years.

Joint replacements are meant to eliminate pain, restore limb alignment, and renew functionality. Many people think that having such operations means giving up an active lifestyle. In fact, the opposite is true. Traditionally, people limited their post-replacement mobility to low-impact activities, but now many patients desire to return to higher-impact sports, such as alpine skiing. I want and expect patients to get moving after I replace their knees and hips, and I allow them to do anything they want—except run. Studies have shown that the level of activity you return to after joint replacement is related to your activity level prior to surgery. If you were active or an athlete prior to surgery, you will return to sport after surgery.

WILL A NEW JOINT GIVE YOU YOUR OLD LIFE BACK?

"I've got to be back on my feet by April so I can train for the drum and bugle corps world championships this summer. I have not missed a competition in 20 years, and if we win we will be four-time world champs." I did not know that adults competed in drum and bugle corps competitions or how serious these events were, but my patient George was eager to teach me. This 54-year-old marcher had torn his ACL (anterior cruciate ligament) as a youth and never had it fixed. Now he had end-stage arthritis on the inside of his knee, and it was preventing him from marching at 80 to 90 steps per minute for hours on end. On top of that, the pain was so great that he could hardly function the day after he worked out. I could tell by talking to George that suggesting an alternative means of exercising was not going to fly. We had six months until the competition, and it usually takes three months to rehab back to sports after a total knee replacement. We had no time to waste.

George worked really hard in therapy, beginning the day after his operation. He walked the hallways of the hospital and kept his eye on the prize as he pushed himself back to full activity. Ultimately, he was able to march at a cadence of 80 to 90 steps per minute all while playing a bugle. After the competition, I received a picture in the mail of George wearing his blue and white competition uniform with the gold medal of victory around his neck. For George, knee replacement was a license for mobility that gave him his life back.

HOW IS JOINT REPLACEMENT DONE?

When cartilage wears down and the bones begin to rub on one another, it causes both pain and deformity. One side of the knee wears out faster than the other, and the bones become lopsided. Most people wear out the inside (medial) portion of the knee joint and the top of the hip joint first. This is why many people become bowlegged as they age.

All joint replacements, therefore, are meant to decrease pain and realign joints so that they are straight again. Joint replacement is performed by making an incision over the involved joint and removing the ends of the bones that no longer have cartilage on them. Special jigs are used to measure and align the cuts made on the ends of the bones to make sure the new joint is anatomically aligned like the natural joint was before arthritis wore it down. Today, doctors use computer navigation in the operating room to more precisely perform this task. The surgical approach to a patient's joint is determined by the surgeon's preference and the patient's anticipated postoperative activity level.

Once all the bone cuts have been made, the ends of the bones are replaced with metal replicas. Prior to surgery, X-rays are measured to make sure that the proper sized implants are available, and during surgery, the surgeon measures to determine what size joint replacement is needed. When the surgeon confirms the proper size and alignment of the implants, they are cemented into place. This is why you can walk on joint replacements immediately.

The implants are made out of cobalt-chrome, ceramic, or titanium alloys and are polished to a highly shiny surface. They reflect light like a polished chrome bumper or a mirror. Between the two polished steel implants, a very tough piece of plastic, called polyethylene or poly, is inserted. The two bone ends move over this poly surface like your natural joint moves over its cartilage.

Rehabilitation after joint replacement surgery can take three to six months, depending on the kind of shape a patient was in prior to surgery. The postoperative results are generally excellent with significant relief of pain and return of function. More than 90 percent of people continue to have good or excellent results more than 10 years after joint replacement. A survey of total joint specialists by the American Association of Hip and Knee Surgeons showed that 95 percent do not restrict their patients' participation in swimming, golfing, walking, cycling, or stair climbing. Truly high-impact sports (such as running) are discouraged, but there remains a lack of scientific evidence to support this recommendation. Several studies show that active people have better results from total joint replacement as a result of better bony ingrowth and fixation of the implants and superior functional strength, balance, endurance, and proprioception.

If you are thinking about having a total joint replacement, the most important word for you right now is *pre-hab*. This means getting in as good shape as you possibly can *before* you have surgery. This will enable you to recover and get out of the hospital faster, perform your exercises better after surgery, and ultimately get back to life sooner. A good place to start getting in shape for joint replacement is with the leg and core exercises you have already learned.

Many active people are opting for partial knee replacements or hip resurfacing instead of total joint replacements when appropriate. In these procedures, less original joint is removed and the implants replace only the portions of the joint most severely affected by arthritis. Although the data is limited, it is very encouraging: In some studies, 93 percent of partial knee recipients returned to pre-op sports.

METAL MEETS THE ROAD

After the American Association of Hip and Knee Surgeons surveyed its members, the group offered the following recommendations on activities for patients who had undergone total joint replacement.

In reality, each surgeon usually determines what his or her patients should do.

Allowed	**Allowed with Experience**	**Not Recommended**
Aerobics	Cross-country skiing	Basketball
Ballroom dancing	Downhill skiing	Football
Bowling	Horseback riding	Running
Golfing	Ice-skating	Soccer
Road cycling	Rowing	Volleyball
Speed walking	Tennis	
Swimming	Weight lifting	
Track cycling		
Walking		

You can find more information about joint replacement at the website of the American Academy of Orthopaedic Surgeons at www.orthoinfo.aaos.org/menus/arthroplasty.cfm and at www.anationinmotion.org.

HOMEWORK

If you have been told that you need a joint replacement, you have homework to do before you sign up. Find the answers to these questions:

- *How many joint replacements does your surgeon do a year?* You want to find a surgeon whose practice is primarily joint replacement.
- *Does your surgeon do her own revision/complication surgery, or does she refer this out?* You want a surgeon who not only performs the primary surgery but will also continue to care for you over the years if you have problems.
- *Will your surgeon send you for pre-hab before surgery?* If your insurance pays for it or if you are willing to invest in this yourself, pre-hab will make a big difference in how strong you feel when you recover.
- *How many days will you be in the hospital?* The typical hospital stay for a knee replacement is three to five days. For a hip replacement, it is one to three days.
- *Will you have inpatient or outpatient rehabilitation after surgery?* For both knee and hip replacements, after you leave the hospital, you may go to an inpatient rehabilitation center for a week or so of intensive physical rehab. If you go straight home from the hospital, you will immediately begin therapy as an out-patient.

- *What kind of blood thinner will you use?* After a knee or hip replacement, it is standard practice to take a blood thinner, in the form of shots or pills, to prevent blood clots in the legs. Blood clots are not common, but they can cause problems if they occur. Blood thinners are typically given for three weeks after surgery.

"It is ironic that humankind has been searching for and developing exotic ways to enhance longevity for millennia, when the longevity factor may literally have been under our noses . . . for millions of years."

—Joseph Maroon, M.D., neurosurgeon and author of *The Longevity Factor*

CHAPTER THIRTEEN

13

It's a Waistline, Not a Wasteline—Your Guide to Smart Nutrition

For many of my masters athletes and adult-onset exercisers, fortifying their bodies and building a better brain through smart nutrition is a big mystery. Every day there seems to be different advice on the best way to feed ourselves for maximum performance—in life and in sport.

When did food get so complicated?

In the first edition of *Fitness After 40*, we spent a lot of time talking about how to fuel the revolution taking place in your body. To maximize performance and minimize injury, you need to be strategic about your mobility and smart about your nutrition. We have overhauled this chapter for this edition, vastly expanding the sections about macronutrients (carbohydrates, protein, and fat) and micronutrients (vitamins and minerals). We also discuss detailed strategies for creating an anti-inflammatory environment in your body and how to be deliberate about supplementing your whole food diet. We also have expanded the section about nutrition for vegetarian and vegan athletes.

MY OWN FITNESS AFTER 40 SMART NUTRITION STORY

While in training, young surgeons never know when they are going to have a minute to eat (or sleep or go to the bathroom either, for that matter), so we eat whatever we have access to—whenever we have access to it. Sometimes it feels like a matter of survival just to grab whatever stale, fatty meal or candy bar is around. As an intern (when I was on the lowest stratum of the totem pole and navigating the most hectic year of my training) and also as a resident, I regularly worked 120 hours per week. Sometimes I would go so far as to console myself over having to be awake and running around the hospital and trauma bay by sneaking up to the cafeteria at 2 A.M. for a cheeseburger and fries. After all, I deserved it, right?

Seven years of this unstrategic, survival-type eating resulted in my slowly gaining 25 pounds. I was far from sedentary—I was running around the hospital 120 hours per week and during that time also ran a marathon—but I was putting trash in, and I got trash out.

When I finished my surgical training and had more control of my time, I stopped the 2 A.M. consolation meals, avoided the eat-whenever-I-can tactic, and ramped up my running. I spent more energy than I took in and the weight fell off. To keep it off and fortify my body toward my best health, I continue my love affair with fresh veggies and make five simple choices every day:

1. No fried foods. Period.
2. No salad dressing or sauce on anything. These are a great way to fatten up otherwise healthy food, as many salad dressings have 100 calories of fat per tablespoon.
3. Limit juice. Most juices contain lots of sugar.
4. Limit even "good" fats. One tablespoon of olive oil has 100 calories.
5. No added sugar or simple carbs; complex carbs only. I break this rule only if I'm training for a race (and then I eat a few more carbs).

Rule Number 5 changed my life last year. Intellectually, I know that high levels of sugar are responsible for many diseases, can exacerbate inflammation and body aches, and contribute to weight gain, but since I prefer the taste of sweet over savory, I fell into the habit of eating dark chocolate each afternoon, cookies whenever, and white pasta often. I was still loyal to Rules 1–4, but my sugar habit was getting out of control. I decided to call it quits on being sweeter on the inside than I was on the outside.

On December 1, 2013, I quit added sugar and simple carbs cold turkey. Literally, I ate cookies one day and none the next.

Initially, it was hard—really hard. I was surprised by how much my body craved sweets and by how strong the triggers were that sent me looking for dark chocolate. No meal that ended with savory on my tongue seemed complete.

The good news is that I persisted and a week, a month, and then several months passed with no added sugar. My taste buds and my body stopped expecting that sweet bonus, and once that happened, I didn't want to go back.

Committing to this single great food choice had two surprise benefits. First, I lost 11 pounds within four weeks without even trying. (This literally meant that I had been consuming 11 pounds of sugar each month!) While losing those pounds was nice (because it put me back to my prepregnancy weight), you know I'm not about the dress size, so it won't surprise you to learn that it was the second benefit that really wowed me.

At the writing of this second edition, I am the 47-year-old mother of a seven-year-old daughter. I'm in shape, but playing on the floor with little ones had caused my joints to ache. I would get up off the floor and feel like I needed to oil my hinges. But when I followed my Rule Number 5 and stopped eating added sugar and simple carbs, all my aching went away. I repeat: *All* my aching away.

My story is not unique. Do you remember the ThermaCare survey I cited in Chapter 11? Participants older than 40 reported that:

- 67 percent suffer from muscle or joint pain weekly
- 73 percent say muscle and joint pain is a bigger annoyance than making sure they remain physically active
- 69 percent claimed they were willing to work through their pain to remain active

For me, making one simple choice—and then receiving the benefit of living in this new, anti-inflamed body—was life changing. *You* can make these simple choices, too.

THE ANTI-INFLAMMATORY DIET

Nutritionists and sports specialists have new awareness about inflammation—how it interferes with athletic performance and how it can be prevented or eased with the right choice of foods. Inflammation can occur without cause, but frequently it is the result of injury during exercise or sports. We all need a small amount of inflammation in our bodies to maintain good health. This is known as acute inflammation. For instance, with an allergic reaction or infection, our bodies are programmed to respond, identifying the infectious or dangerous substance and repairing any resulting damage.

When our bodies are working smoothly and properly, the pro-inflammatory compounds that are part of this response are released easily and efficiently, as needed. Once the threat has been addressed, our bodies return to a balanced state. However, when inflammation occurs without obvious cause or when the inflammatory response is overactive, the inflammation can become chronic. This not only affects athletic ability but can also lead to heart problems and autoimmune disorders, such as arthritis and allergies.

Recently, many new anti-inflammatory diets have been released. While these diets vary greatly in terms of menu advice, all are based on the concept that constant irritation leads to a variety of maladies. Such diets are good for general health but also help decrease an athlete's susceptibility to inflammation before, during, and after exercise or sports. In general, anti-inflammatory diets are not designed for weight loss, although if you follow these regimens, you probably will lose weight.

The following lists are a compilation of the anti-inflammatory foods and vitamins presented by researchers in the field, including those from Norway, the land of super-athletes. Of course, you have your own likes and dislikes, as well as individual athletic goals. So feel free to choose from these lists as it suits you.

Anti-Inflammatory Foods

Try to avoid foods that may trigger inflammation. These include processed carbohydrates, such as white flour and white sugar, as well as saturated and trans fats, such as those found in fried foods. Avoid cooking oils, such as sunflower and cottonseed oils; full-fat dairy, such as butter and cheese; red meat and processed meat, such as salamis and sausages; alcohol; and artificial food additives. I recommend the following anti-inflammatory foods:

- ***Vegetables***. Broccoli, cauliflower, and spinach are high in anti-inflammatory nutrients. Mushrooms increase immunity levels. Onions are a good source of quercetin, a powerful antioxidant. (Antioxidants protect against harmful substances, called "free radicals," in your body that can damage DNA and lead to cancer and other diseases.) Additional vegetables that reputedly reduce inflammation include brussels sprouts, cabbage, green beans, kelp, leeks, olives, turnip greens, spinach, and sweet potatoes.
- ***Fruits***. Apple skins contain quercetin; papayas and pineapples are high in healing substances; and berries have antioxidants to calm inflammation. Other anti-inflammatory fruits include grapefruits, guavas, kiwis, limes, melons, and oranges.

- ***Herbs and spices***. The following add-ins are rich in phytochemicals, which are inflammation suppressants: Turmeric has recently been reported to have an anti-inflammatory effect similar to medications such as cortisone. Ginger and garlic have long been used in folk medicines to treat internal inflammation. Other herbs and spices that calm inflammation include basil, black pepper, chives, cilantro, cinnamon, cloves, oregano, parsley, and rosemary.
- ***Oils***. Olive oil is generally thought to be one of the best oils, although not all specialists believe it. Eucalyptus oil is another pure oil said to help fight chronic inflammation.
- ***Nuts and seeds***. Almonds, flaxseed, hazelnuts, peanuts, pecans, pine seeds, sesame seeds, sunflower seeds, and walnuts are all excellent anti-inflammatory foods.

Anti-Inflammatory Vitamins

In addition to whole foods, individual vitamins provide numerous anti-inflammatory benefits. The following are some of the best.

- ***Vitamin A***. This is an antioxidant that also has anti-inflammatory effects. A University of Oslo researcher, Ingrid Benedicte Moss Kolseth, found that a derivative of Vitamin A given to patients undergoing surgery for colon cancer resulted in less pain and suppressed inflammatory response before and after surgery. Vitamin A is commonly found in liver, whole milk, and some fortified foods. Beta-carotene, a provitamin (a metabolically inactive substance that is converted in the body to an active vitamin) found in carrots and many colorful vegetables, can be converted to Vitamin A in the body.
- ***Vitamin B6***. This member of the B vitamin family is plentiful in foods such as beef, fish, turkey, and vegetables. Because

Vitamin B6 is water-soluble, your body needs to restock it daily through diet.

- ***Vitamin C***. This plays a role in protecting your joints, boosting your immune system, and relieving inflammation throughout your entire body. Your body absorbs and uses Vitamin C immediately and excretes any excess, which is why it is important to consume foods rich in Vitamin C throughout the day.

- ***Vitamin D***. This is essential for the absorption of calcium and phosphorus and for bone formation. If you have unexplained muscle pain or weakness or low calcium balance, you may need more Vitamin D, but check with your healthcare provider. A deficiency in Vitamin D has also been linked to a number of inflammatory diseases, including arthritis and inflammatory bowel disease (IBD). Vitamin D is present in oily fish, eggs, and dairy products in variable amounts. It is not found in plant foods. Vitamin D is also manufactured by your skin when you are exposed to sunlight. Getting Vitamin D in this way is usually enough to meet your body's requirements, but eating fortified foods ensures that you get amounts adequate for an athletic lifestyle.

- ***Vitamin E***. This comes in several different forms of natural mixed tocopherols (a class of organic chemical compounds). Vitamin E is another antioxidant with anti-inflammatory properties. Common food sources include nuts, seeds, and green leafy vegetables.

- ***Vitamin K***. This is found in green vegetables, such as asparagus, broccoli, kale, and spinach, and is best known for its role in helping blood clot, but research is finding that it may have other benefits, too.

SHAPE UP AND EAT WELL

Do you know your body shape? You are either a "pear," which means you carry your extra weight around your hips, or you are an "apple," which means you carry it around your waist. It is better to be a pear than an apple. Those of you who inherited apple-shaped bodies are at increased risk for overall health problems, such as diabetes, heart disease, high blood pressure, and obesity. You were born this way but you can decrease your health risk by minimizing your fat storage. As long as you avoid excess weight, being an apple doesn't put you at special risk. Ideally, men's waists should be less than 40 inches and women's less than 35.

Gaining and losing weight is neither a complicated nor a mystical goal that few can grasp. It is a numbers game. Unless you have a real medical problem, such as a thyroid dysfunction or diabetes, to lose weight you have to take in fewer calories than you expend. Did I hear the crowd say "Duh!"? It sounds simple, and it is, yet more than two-thirds of us don't have a handle on how to consume only what we need each day. In fact, weight gain is often such a gradual process that we don't realize it is happening until we've put on 10 or 20 pounds. And, truth be told, our modern society tempts us to consume more than we need on a daily, perhaps even hourly, basis. For example, 20 years ago, a 16-ounce cup of coffee had 45 calories. Today's 16-ounce cup of gourmet flavored coffee has 350 calories. It takes you about three miles (about an hour) of walking to burn the 350 calories in that fancy cup of joe. Is it worth it?

When sedentary people begin one of my exercise programs, I have their body composition measured. We are able to tell exactly what percentage of their body is lean and what percentage is fat. One session included 89 sedentary people who were

Table 4. The Risk of Developing Health Problems According to Body Mass Index (BMI) and Waist Circumference

Rating	BMI	Obesity class	Men: Waist < 40 in. Women: Waist < 35 in.	Men: Waist < 40 in. Women: Waist < 35 in.
Underweight	< 18.5	—	—	—
Normal	18.5–24.9	—	—	Central obesity is a health risk
Overweight	25–29.9	—	Increased	High
Obese	30–34.9	I	High	Very High
	35–39.9	II	Very High	Very High
Extreme	> 40	III	Extremely High	Extremely High

just beginning to exercise. The average body fat for the women in this group was 51 percent; for the men, it was 41 percent. A healthy body fat is 18–25 percent. (Table 4 presents information on body shape and the risk of developing health problems.)

These people looked like average citizens. They knew they had a few pounds to lose but would never have guessed how much extra they were actually carrying around. They were surprised and taken aback by their bodies. It is easy not to notice what is happening to you.

If you suspect that you need to lose a few pounds, start reading the labels on the foods you eat. Notice what the manufacturer considers to be a serving size and how many calories that amount contains. (You may discover that manufacturers' idea of serving sizes is much smaller than yours.) You will be surprised by how quickly the calories add up.

Healthy, sustainable weight loss is approximately one pound per week. This means burning 500 calories more than you take in each day. When you think about it, that is not really too much of a sacrifice. It means cutting out the morning Danish, not drinking two cans of soda while on break, or walking right past the candy machine. Are you saying "blah, blah, blah . . . I have heard this before!"? Yes, you probably have—and yet, you may not be in control of your intake.

As I told you earlier in this chapter, I love sweets and have to make a conscious decision every time I pass our vending machines. When I finally decided to cut added sugar and simple carbs from my diet, it was really tough. But after being good for several days, I talked myself through the urge: "Vonda, you went two days without that Snickers and didn't shrivel up and die. Walk on by!" After a while, I got to where I didn't want to break my streak of good behavior.

Now that we've talked about what your body *doesn't* need, let's talk about what it *does*.

MACRONUTRIENTS

Medical literature is full of studies that recognize the importance of proper nutrition and how it connects with exercise performance. What you put in your body not only affects your overall health and weight but your recovery time and performance.

Athletes of any level, independent of age, must consume adequate dietary energy to offset energy expenditure, maintain body weight and health, and maximize training effort. Too much in and you get fat. Too little in and you lose muscle and bone (because, when needed, the body uses itself as a resource/storehouse), increase fatigue, and become prone to injury and illness. But how much is enough?

The rest of this chapter outlines what your body needs as fuel. For some, this is all new information; for others, perhaps a quick review. Alert: This chapter is *not* a diet plan. There are thousands of books out there about dieting. I do not advocate dieting or being austere with yourself. I think this just makes people obsess about what foods they are not eating. Instead, I advocate knowing what your body needs and being smart about what you do eat. I will never tell you not to taste the chocolate cake—I will simply advise you not to do it all the time.

You are reading this book because you have decided you want to be the best you can be. The key to this is knowing what are the right foods at the right time for you. After the age of 40, as you know, you are not the same physically as you were. Also, there is a lot of conflicting and potentially harmful information out there. Therefore, you should get clearance from your health-care provider before you change your diet or opt for supplements.

Let's first take an in-depth look at the macronutrients, starting with protein.

Protein

My patients often ask: "How much protein do I really need?" "More protein" is the advice often given if you are into strength-building sports or exercise regimes or if you are just aging. It is true that, if you are an athlete, you need more protein than a less active person, but you don't have to spend your money on special and (usually expensive) protein supplements or big, protein-laced meals. Protein alone will not build your muscles. If you take in more protein and carbohydrates than you need, your body will store the overload as fat tissue. Furthermore, recent research has found that if you eat too many high-protein foods and take protein supplements, you may risk kidney damage, loss of calcium from bones, and dehydration.

There are no specific recommendations on protein intake for older athletes—or older sedentary people, for that matter. Several studies do show that the Recommended Dietary Allowance (RDA) for protein may not be adequate for sustaining and building muscle for aging athletes. If you exercise or weight train and don't ingest enough protein, your body will use itself—your own muscles—as a protein source, resulting in muscle atrophy and loss of fat-free body mass.

The predominant role of protein for exercise is to repair the microdamage that occurs to muscle. A small amount of protein, about 5 percent of our daily intake, is used to fuel exercise. The RDA for protein is 0.8 grams for every kilogram of body weight (1 kilogram is about 2.2 pounds). This means that the average 176-pound man needs to eat 64 grams of protein per day. An ounce of fish or meat has approximately 7 grams of protein.

PROTEIN IN COMMON FOODS

The following list will help you keep track of your protein intake.

Beans/Nuts

- Almonds (1/4 cup): 8 grams
- Most beans (1/2 cup): 7–10 grams
- Peanut butter (2 tablespoons): 8 grams
- Peanuts (1/4 cup): 9 grams
- Pumpkin seeds (1/4 cup): 19 grams

Breads/Cereals/Grains

- 3 grams per serving (a slice of bread, a half cup of cereal, or a half cup of grain)

Chicken

- Breast: 30 grams per 3.5 ounces
- Drumstick: 11 grams per ounce
- Thigh: 10 grams per ounce
- Wing: 6 grams per ounce

Eggs/Dairy Products

- Large egg: 6 grams
- Milk (1 cup): 8 grams
- Yogurt (1 cup): 8–12 grams

Fish

- 22 grams per 3.5 ounces

Pork

- Bacon (1 slice): 3 grams
- Chop: 22 grams per 3 ounces
- Ham: 19 grams per 3 ounces

Red Meat

- 7 grams per 3 ounces

Male endurance athletes require a daily maximum of 1.2–1.4 grams per kilogram of body weight; those engaged in strength training require 1.6–1.7 grams per kilogram of body weight per day to accumulate and maintain muscles. This higher requirement is needed to provide amino acids, or protein building blocks, for the repair of exercise-induced muscle damage, the buildup of lean tissue mass, and the use of protein as an energy source during exercise. (Note that there are no data for women.) Eating a high-protein diet or taking supplements that provide more than these levels is unlikely to increase muscle mass further. There is a limit to the rate that you can build muscle.

According to the Academy of Nutrition and Dietetics, the proteins you eat are involved in building and maintaining your body tissues. As an energy source, proteins are equivalent to carbohydrates in providing 4 calories per gram. Proteins also perform a major structural role in the formation of enzymes, hormones, and various body fluids and secretions. Proteins participate in the transport of some fats, vitamins, and minerals and help maintain your body's homeostasis—the stable state of healthy functioning.

Carbohydrates

Carbohydrates (carbs) have been given a bad name mainly because of best-selling books written by doctors and other nutrition gurus who believe the key to losing weight is to take in less sugars and starches. They are right to a point, but since you are dedicated to your fitness after 40, you need a sufficient amount of carbohydrates (more than your couch potato friends).

Your body converts the sugars and starches in carbohydrates to energy (as glucose) or stores it in your liver (as glycogen). Carbohydrates in the form of glycogen are the fuels that enable you to exercise. Therefore, if you hope to train consistently, you must eat adequate carbs each day.

A high-carbohydrate meal before exercise increases the fuel available for the exercising muscles, which provides benefit during both prolonged endurance exercise and high-intensity exercise. An overnight fast depletes the glycogens stored in the liver and can contribute to light-headedness and the early onset of fatigue. Starting any exercise session hungry or light-headed keeps you from performing your best.

If you are in a hurry or are worried about your weight, eat a small high-carbohydrate snack (a banana, a bagel, cereal, a vegan "energy bar") about an hour and a half before you exercise or drink a glass of a fluid-replacement beverage about 10 minutes prior.

The cells of your body use circulating glucose to make energy at rest and during exercise. Not only do your cells need carbs but your brain is entirely dependent on carbs for energy. Carbs help maintain blood glucose during exercise and restore muscle glycogen during rest and recovery from exercise. The recommended daily intake is a minimum of 130 grams, or 45–65 percent of daily calories for adults, independent of age or activity level. This is the minimum needed for your brain to function. It is recommended that athletes consume 6–10 grams of carbs for every kilogram of body weight per day. For example, a male athlete weighing 70 kilograms (154 pounds) needs 420 grams of carbs per day to fuel his activity. If you are on a low-calorie diet (fewer than 2,000 calories per day), it may be difficult to achieve the recommended 6 grams of carbs per kilogram of weight each day. On a 2,000-calorie-a-day diet, adult women should consume between 160 and 200 grams of carbohydrates a day. The majority should be in the form of less-refined, less-processed foods with a low glycemic (blood sugar) load.

The following tips can help you strike the right carb/calorie balance:

- Reduce your consumption of foods made with white flour and sugar, especially bread and packaged snack foods (including chips and pretzels).
- Eat more whole grains, such as brown rice and bulgur wheat, in which the grain is intact or in a few large pieces. These are preferable to products made with whole wheat flour, which have roughly the same glycemic index as white flour products.
- Eat more beans, winter squashes, and sweet potatoes.
- Cook pasta al dente and eat it in moderation.
- Avoid products made with high-fructose corn syrup.

Age does not alter the role of carbs in generating energy, and older athletes continue to be able to store ingested carbs as a source of energy production during exercise. If you plan to exercise an hour or more, it is recommended that you take in 30–60 grams of carbs, as either food or beverage. This is the purpose of all those nutrition bars and gel packs. Try them out at home before you hit the road or gym because they can sometimes cause stomach upset or diarrhea.

After hard exercise (more than 90 minutes), recovery is optimal with a carb intake afterward. This should consist of 1.5 grams of carbs per kilogram of body weight. An additional carb feeding two hours later helps restore muscle glycogen storage. These recommendations are for aging athletes who train hard and frequently. If you are a recreational athlete and race once in a while, you do not have to worry about recovering with carbs.

Most runners are more concerned with their training than with their diet, but Ernst Albin Hansen, an associate professor at the Department of Health Science and Technology at Aalborg

University in Denmark, says it is possible to shave 11 minutes off your marathon time—with no extra training. You just need to consume the right amount of carbohydrates during the race.

Fat

Fat is not all bad. Despite its bad rap, fat provides energy and is the essential element of cell membranes. Fat also provides Vitamins E, A, and D. There is no RDA for total fat, but a daily intake with 20–35 percent of energy from fat provides adequate oomph while preventing the risk of chronic disease that occurs when fat intake is too high. Lower levels do not enhance physical performance.

How your body uses fat for energy depends upon the intensity and duration of your exercise. If you rest or do low- or moderate-intensity exercise, fat is your primary fuel source. As you increase the intensity of your exercise, your body uses more carbs for fuel. For continuous activities of three to four hours, make sure that the glycogen stores in your muscles and liver are at a maximum. Consider taking carbohydrates (in the form of carbohydrate solutions) during the event. The current recommendation is a 6–8 percent glucose solution.

On a 2,000-calorie-a-day diet, 600 calories can come from fat—that is, about 67 grams. This should be in a ratio of 1:2:1 of saturated to monounsaturated to polyunsaturated fat.

The following tips can help you strike the right balance with your fat intake:

- Reduce your intake of saturated fat by eating less butter, cream, high-fat cheese, chicken with skin, fatty meats, and products made with palm kernel oil.

- Use extra-virgin olive oil as your main cooking oil. If you want a neutral-tasting oil, use expeller-pressed, organic canola oil. Organic, high-oleic, expeller-pressed sunflower and safflower oils are also acceptable.
- Avoid regular safflower and sunflower oils, corn oil, cottonseed oil, and mixed vegetable oils.
- Avoid margarine, vegetable shortening, and all products listing them as ingredients. Strictly avoid all products made with partially hydrogenated oils of any kind.
- Include avocados and nuts (especially almonds, cashews, and walnuts) and nut butters made from these nuts in your diet.
- For omega-3 fatty acids, eat salmon (preferably fresh or frozen wild or canned sockeye); sardines packed in water or olive oil; herring; black cod (sablefish, butterfish); omega-3 fortified eggs; and hemp seeds and flaxseeds (preferably freshly ground). You can also take a fish oil supplement (look for products that provide both EPA and DHA, in a convenient daily dosage of 2–3 grams).

WANT TO LOSE BODY FAT?

Here's the secret: Eat!

Your body has developed a variety of strategies to store and hold on to calories more efficiently if it doesn't know when your next meal will be. Skipping meals makes your body think it is starving and activates all the defenses designed to protect itself from true starvation. Let's talk numbers. When women eat less than 800 to 1,200 calories and men eat less than 1,200 to 1,800 calories per day, their metabolisms slow down, and their bodies use their own muscle as fuel.

A sure way to increase your metabolism is to increase your muscle-to-fat ratio. In other words, you should develop your "C" (carry a load). After all, muscle takes more energy to live than fat. Another way to increase your metabolism is to eat small meals every three hours. This approach works for several reasons:

- Food digestion itself burns a lot of calories.
- A steady stream of healthy mini-meals prevents desperate vending machine binges.
- Small meals control fat storage.
- Nutrients are effectively utilized.
- Complex carbohydrates plus lean proteins and healthy fats stabilize your blood glucose and insulin levels, preventing the post-meal energy crash.

Fluids

Water is *the* most important factor in sports nutrition. You can't manufacture it, so you have to replace the water you lose from sweat and urination. If you take away only one pointer from this section, it should be: *Don't trust your thirst*. Here's why.

The adult body is 50–70 percent water. The leaner you are, the greater your percentage is, since muscle contains more than 80 percent water while fat has less than 30 percent. Disturbances in water and electrolyte balance affect us at all levels—from systemic to cellular—and prevent our ability to exercise.

Hot and dry will hurt you, as even modest dehydration (less than 2 percent fluid loss) can affect athletic performance. When you are dehydrated, you sweat at a slower rate and therefore cannot cool your body as effectively. Overheating impairs cardiovascular function and strains the heart. As you lose water, you experience a linear rise in your core body temperature, with every liter of water loss resulting in an increase of .06°F (0.3°C).

Age-related changes amplify this effect. With age, we have an altered thirst mechanism. Our kidneys can become less efficient, we waste water more, and our blood vessels are less flexible and dilate less. These, in turn, reduce our ability to release heat through our skin.

You should drink at least 2 quarts (the equivalent of 8 cups or 1.89 liters) of water every day. Drink a lot of water during and after a sports event. When you work out or compete, especially in hot weather, try to closely match the amount of fluid you need with the amount you lose in sweat. As mentioned above, do not trust your thirst. Your thirst mechanism is not strong enough to stimulate adequate fluid intake during exercise. You must therefore have a fluid plan for optimal performance. This plan should be divided into pre-hydration before exercise, hydration during exercise, and re-hydration after exercise.

- ***Pre-hydration***. It is easier to prevent dehydration than to catch up during exercise. The American College of Sports Medicine recommends consuming 500mL (milliliters), or 16.9 ounces—the size of an average water bottle—of fluid one to two hours prior to exercise to make sure you are ready to exercise and give yourself time to get rid of the extra fluid.

- ***Hydration***. Hydration is meant to prevent or minimize dehydration during exercise. There is no evidence that you need carb drinks if you are going to exercise for less than one hour; water is enough. When exercising one hour or more, however, you should take carb drinks. This prevents the muscle fatigue that usually occurs with exercise lasting more than one hour. Carb drinks should have a 4–8 percent concentration, since a concentration of greater than 10 percent causes fluid to be drawn into the gut (water always moves to the place where its concentration is lowest), which not only removes the fluid from the areas in your body that need it the most but could cause diarrhea.

The term *gastric emptying* refers to how fast the fluid you drink is used. To maximize fluid usage, you should keep your stomach as full of water as you can tolerate without vomiting—usually about one bottle containing 16.9 ounces (500mL). Regular exercise does not appear to alter gastric emptying; high-intensity exercise (at 80 percent or more of maximum effort) inhibits gastric emptying. During exercise, sweat should be replaced by fluid intake of 6–12 ounces (roughly 177–355mL) every 20 minutes. Begin drinking early during your exercise; it is better to prevent dehydration than to play catch-up. This is easier said than done when you are focusing on exercise or a race. It is not uncommon for an athlete to become so dehydrated that he loses 4.4–6.6 pounds (2–3 kilograms) of body weight during a race from water loss alone.

The early signs of dehydration are subtle and may be easy to miss. They include dark yellow urine, dry mouth, headaches, weakness, irritability, and cramping. When dehydration progresses, you may not urinate or produce tears or you may experience fainting, rapid heart rate, low blood pressure, and changes in clarity of thought.

- ***Re-hydration***. After exercise, you will probably be thirsty. Even if you are not, drink anyway. It is common for us to dehydrate our body weight by 2–6 percent during exercise, especially in the heat. For every pound that you sweat off, you should drink 16–23 ounces (473–680mL) after an exercise session. Avoid caffeine or alcohol (even if your race is sponsored by Bud Light). You will know that you have hydrated back up to normal when your urine is clear or pale. If it remains dark yellow, drink up.

ARE YOU A SALTY SWEATER?

During my pre-performance physical of Mike, one of my PRIMA athletes, he mentioned that he often got a lot of cramps after a long workout despite the fact that he drank adequate fluids and ate bananas (the supposed cramp prevention food) like they were going out of style. After further questioning, he mentioned that at the end of a marathon or on a really hot day, his skin felt like gritty sandpaper covered in salt. Mike is a salty sweater: He loses a lot of salt through his skin while sweating. Although many of us are of the mindset that we need to limit our salt intake (to decrease our chances of high blood pressure), when we sweat like this, we can actually have too little salt in our bodies. This can lead to cramps—even if you eat a lot of bananas. (Bananas give you potassium but not a lot of salt.)

Mike met with PRIMA's nutritionist, Leslie Bonci, and she evaluated his diet and fluid intake. She discovered that he was not taking in enough salt (sodium) to replace the salt he lost during exercise. This was leading to his frequent cramps. She recommended he add a little salt to his diet with pretzels, soy sauce, and Worcestershire sauce, and miraculously, his cramps decreased. Leslie also recommends drinking sports drinks during long workouts to replace the electrolytes (salt, potassium, etc.) you lose.

HYDRATION RECOMMENDATIONS

The following recommendations on hydration are from the American College of Sports Medicine:

- Eat and drink a balanced and adequate diet in the 24 hours prior to an event, including the meal prior to exercise.
- Drink 16.9 ounces (500mL) of water within the two hours prior to exercise to provide adequate hydration and give you time to urinate the excess. (Nothing kills a workout—or worse, a race—than having to stop to pee.)
- During a race, begin drinking early and continue drinking to prevent dehydration. It is easier to stay on top of it than try to catch up.
- Fluids should be cooler than the outside air (55–72°F; 12.7–22.2°C) and flavored, so they go down more easily.
- If you are exercising less than an hour, you do not need to replace carbs and electrolytes. Water is fine.
- During intense exercise (lasting longer than an hour), replace your electrolytes and your carbs (at a rate of 30–60 grams of carbs per hour). This is equal to one of those glucose packs. More practically, this can be achieved by drinking 600–1200mL each hour (or one to two 20-ounce bottles) of a 4–8 percent carb drink.
- The replacement fluid should contain 0.5–0.7 grams per liter of sodium to promote fluid retention and prevent excess loss of sodium from excess fluid intake.

Micronutrients

Micronutrients are nutrients, including vitamins and minerals, that are needed in only small amounts. Regular exercise may increase our need for vitamins and minerals, which serve a variety of roles, including energy production, synthesis of hemoglobin (the part of blood that carries oxygen), bone health, immune function, muscle building after exercise, and protection from oxidative damage. (Oxidative damage occurs because our cells produce substances called free radicals when working or harmed, and these hurt the surrounding cells.) As with macronutrients, insufficient intake of micronutrients affects your daily life and athletic performance.

Most of the time, we can get adequate amounts of vitamins and minerals from our diets if we are following the RDAs. The Academy of Nutrition and Dietetics states that "no vitamin or mineral supplement should be required if an athlete is consuming adequate energy from a variety of foods to maintain body weight." But coupling exercise with a restrictive diet, a diet that leaves out food groups, or a diet that includes empty calories may result in insufficient vitamin and mineral intake. Age may also present a special challenge for absorbing enough vitamins and minerals because of low-energy intake, impaired absorption, chronic medical problems, and medications. Table 5 presents information on important vitamins and minerals for aging athletes.

Table 5. Important Vitamins and Minerals for the Aging Athlete

Vitamin/ Mineral	Function	Dietary Intake	Differences/Recommendations for Aging Athletes/Exercisers
Riboflavin	Energy metabolism	Women = 1.1 mg Men = 1.3 mg	Increased requirement for female endurance athletes. High carb diet may increase bacterial synthesis and decrease dietary need.
Vitamin B6	Amino acid and glycogen metabolism	Women = 1.5 mg Men = 1.7 mg	Age increases requirement. Inadequate B6 compromises immunity. Some nutritionists suggest increased levels to 2.0 mg/day.
Vitamin B12	Nucleic acid metabolism; prevents anemia; required for RBC (red blood cell) synthesis	Women = 2.4 ug Men = 2.4 ug	Atrophic gastritis, common with aging, prevents B12 absorption and increases the risk of anemia. Vegetarians require 2.8 ug since B12 is found only in animal foods.
Folate	Amino acid metabolism; nucleic acid and RBC synthesis; prevents anemia	Women = 400 ug Men = 400 ug	Atrophic gastritis, common with aging, prevents folic acid absorption and increases the risk of anemia.
Vitamin D	Bone health; enhances calcium absorption; modulates immune function	Women 50–70 = 10 ug Women > 70 = 15 ug Men 50–70 = 10 ug Men > 70 = 15 ug	Older skin is less able to synthesis vitamin D, which is a steroid hormone that is produced less after menopause. Must supplement.
Vitamin E	Antioxidant: prevents oxidative damage	Women = 15 mg Men = 15 mg	Protects against cataracts, heart disease. Extra may not be necessary for athletes but some studies suggest increased intake to 100 mg for endurance sports.
Calcium	Bone health; blood clotting; muscle contraction; nerve conduction	Women = 1200 mg Men = 1200 mg	Protects against stress fractures. Atrophic gastritis decreases absorption. Lost via sweat.
Iron	RBC production; prevents anemia	Women = 8 mg Men = 8 mg	Iron stores increase with age so supplementation may be less necessary.

Adapted with permission from W. W. Campbell and R. A. Geik, "Nutritional Considerations for the Older Athlete," *Nutrition* 20(7–8): 603–608 (2004).

NUTRITIONAL SUPPLEMENTS

Since the first recognition that nutrition matters in achieving peak performance, a multimillion-dollar market has developed focusing on the athlete's and exerciser's desire to be the best. A huge number of nutritional aids, herbal supplements, and diet pills claim to quickly enhance performance or fitness. By some estimations, there are currently more than 800 medications under development for "anti-aging" uses. The supplement market is not well regulated, and many of the claims made on bottle labels or infomercials are not supported by sound research. In other words, be careful what you put in your mouth. If you want to be the best you can be, eat a balanced diet, hydrate, and minimize severe weight loss.

Another hot topic today is the role of testosterone and growth hormone supplementation for age-related muscle decline. Both of these hormones occur naturally in the body and decline with age. The sections below detail some of the science behind popular and controversial anti-aging drugs and supplements with the goal of clarifying the good, the bad, and the simply unsubstantiated.

Testerone

Testosterone is well studied as an effective performance-enhancing supplement for athletes. It is less well studied for anti-aging. Our fascination with testosterone began in the 1800s when Arnold A. Berthold at the Göttingen Zoo in Germany castrated roosters and found they stopped fighting, crowing, and being interested in hens. When their testicles were reimplanted into their abdomen, they regained their "natural vigor." Subsequently, Charles-Édouard Brown-Séquard proceeded to self-inject "testicular extracts" and reported a return of his own "old powers." After testosterone was synthesized in 1935, it was quickly adopted as a performance enhancer.

A significant number of men—20 percent of 60-year-olds and 70 percent of 70-year-olds—have low testosterone and are considered "hypogonadal." This results in a decline in sexual activity, a reduction of lean muscle mass, and an increase in falls, fractures, depression, and cognitive failure. Ultimately, low testosterone can make men frail.

Many studies demonstrate restoration of libido and erectile function with testosterone supplementation. Importantly, testosterone increases cognitive function, enhances verbal and visual memory, and elevates mood. Testosterone supplementation for hypogonadism also improves functional physical performance and bone density in older men. More than 29 randomized clinical trials studying more than 1,000 older men found that testosterone decreases bone fat by 6 percent over six months and enhances the effect of exercise on strength. None of these studies raised circulating testosterone to hyper levels; rather, they raised low testosterone levels to normal physiologic levels and, in so doing, found that they returned the "vital" functions of their subjects.

Whether or not to test and treat hypogonadism is a decision each man must carefully consider. Your primary care physician can help you understand the specific risks this treatment may present for you, including a heightened risk of prostate cancer.

Resveratrol

Why don't French women get fat despite a diet of red wine and delicious sauces? The so-called "French paradox" puzzled scientists until the discovery that the skins of red grapes—most specifically, Pinot Noir—contained resveratrol, which activates the Sirtuin 1 gene, which encodes specific proteins. This activation stops programmed cell death and reverses the detrimental cell pathways of a high-fat diet. In 2006, *Nature* published a report that resveratrol may stop cancer cells, prevent or reverse coronary artery disease, and break down beta-amyloid (the component of plaques that characterize Alzheimer's disease). You would need to drink about 2,000 glasses of Pinot Noir a day in order to achieve the levels of resveratrol needed to obtain these physiologic advantages—not an option. Resveratrol is considered a supplement, not a drug, and therefore is unregulated. If you take resveratrol, make sure you know what you are getting.

Growth Hormone

Despite what you read in the paper (and the word of Rocky Balboa), more than 30 high-quality randomized clinical trials exist on growth hormone supplementation. In a meta-analysis of these studies, growth hormone was found to cause a very mild change in body composition through fat loss and muscle gain of 7 percent. There was no increase in muscle strength or bone mineral density.

The medical literature uniformly denounces growth hormone as a performance enhancer and cites a long list of complications caused by its ingestion, including soft tissue edema, joint pain, breast swelling in men and women, and new-onset diabetes. In addition, it is currently a felony to prescribe or take growth hormone and the penalty can include five years in prison and up to a $250,000 fine.

Creatine

Creatine and its derivative, phosphocreatine (a high-energy compound necessary for muscle contraction), occur naturally in the human body. Some people take synthetic forms of creatine in hopes of enhancing muscle performance. After it is ingested, stores of both creatine and phosphocreatine in the muscle can increase.

Researchers at the Ohio State University found that male swimmers who took creatine for two weeks improved their time by an average of 0.73 seconds during a 50-meter swim. However, female swimmers in the same study did not appear to benefit from creatine supplementation. While this study suggested that taking supplemental creatine does have a cumulative effect, Nicole Leenders, coauthor of the study, hesitates to recommend it to athletes—elite or otherwise

WHEN TO EAT

The timing of meals can enhance athletic performance. For sustained calorie regulation and blood glucose (sugar) control, it is best to eat small meals throughout the day. If you are trying to use 500 calories more than you take in each day, it is best not to skip eating. Your body doesn't know you are trying to lose weight and simply recognizes the deprivation, thinks it is starving, and shifts into a storage mode.

On the other hand, eating sugar or honey just before an event does not provide any extra energy for the event. It can take about 30 minutes for the sugar to enter the bloodstream, so it does not provide immediate energy. This practice may also lead to dehydration because water is needed to absorb the sugar into the cells. Furthermore, sugar eaten before an event may hinder performance because it triggers a surge of insulin. The insulin causes a sharp drop in blood sugar level in about 30 minutes. Competing when the blood sugar level is low leads to fatigue, nausea, and dehydration.

A diet where 70 percent of calories come from carbohydrates for three days prior to the event is sometimes helpful for endurance athletes. However, water retention is often associated with carbohydrate loading. This may cause stiffness in the muscles and sluggishness early in the event. A three-day regimen minimizes this effect.

A small, pre-exercise carbohydrate-rich snack within one hour of training has been shown to enhance performance. This little energy boost should be low in fat and fiber and contain a moderate amount of protein. If you are a morning exerciser, try one bottle of sports drink prior to exercising since fasting through the night leaves your liver stores of fuel low. The first time you try this, make sure you are near a bathroom, since some people tolerate food coupled with exercise better than others.

If you are into endurance exercise that lasts three to four hours, your body will love carbs while you are exercising. Thirty to 60 grams of carbs per hour will extend your performance if you start taking them early in your race or workout.

The Academy of Nutrition and Dietetics recommends that runners supplement their natural energy stores by consuming 60 grams of carbohydrates per hour during a marathon. This is equivalent to an hourly intake of approximately three energy gels, which are carbohydrates in viscous form and are rapidly absorbed in the body.

After a long workout, take your first carb boost in the first 30 minutes of recovery and then every two hours for four to six hours. This results in a higher stored glycogen level than if you delayed eating for two hours.

If you are timing full meals on the day of your competition, you can usually figure that it takes about four to five hours to completely digest a normal-sized meal. Some athletes find that they are more nervous before competing, and anxiety usually slows the digestive process. Allowing more time before exercising, eating a lower-fat meal, doing relaxation techniques, or even trying liquid meals (a fruit smoothie made of low-fat yogurt blended with fruit, or an instant breakfast drink made with non-fat milk) have helped athletes with nerves.

STRATEGIC EATING

Strategically eating begins like strategically exercising—by making small changes daily. You need to think about what you eat and slowly begin to change your diet as necessary. Now that we have talked about your exercise-output connection, the important role your mind plays in facing your future, and your nutritional input, let's get down to the nitty-gritty of thinking about individual meals.

KEEP AN EYE ON PORTION SIZE

What is the difference between portions and servings? A "portion" is the amount of any given food you choose to eat—whether for dinner, snack, or other eating occasion. Portions, of course, can be bigger or smaller than the recommended food servings.

A "serving" is a unit of measure used to describe the amount of food recommended from each food group. It is the amount of food listed in the Nutrition Facts panel on packaged food or the amount of food recommended in the Dietary Guidelines released by the U.S. government.

For example, six to 11 servings of whole grains are recommended daily. A recommended serving of whole grains would be one slice of bread or a half cup of rice or pasta. (Download the Serving Size Card at the website hp2010.nhlbihin.net/portion/servingcard7.pdf for more examples of recommended serving sizes.) People often confuse the recommendation to mean six to 11 portions with no regard to size. It is *not* six to 11 portions where one portion could mean a large bowl of pasta rather than a half cup. Keep an eye on portion size to see how your portions compare with the recommended amounts.

Check out the sample menus at www.nhlbi.nih.gov/health/educational/lose_wt/menuplanner.html to see examples of appropriate portions and serving sizes. The sample menus can help you create reduced-calorie meal plans. These items use the servings recommended by the Academy of Nutrition and Dietetics. The servings recommended by that group may differ from the Nutrition Facts panel and the Dietary Guidelines. See the Food Exchange Lists at www.nhlbi.nih.gov/health/public/heart/obesity/lose_wt/fd_exch.htm to give yourself more choices.

Breakfast

These simple breakfast choices may work for you:

- Yogurt with graham crackers
- Bowl of cereal with low-fat milk
- Low-fat granola bar
- Fig Newtons and a glass of low-fat milk
- Bagel with a slice of low-fat cheese
- Fruit smoothie made with non-fat yogurt
- Steel-cut oatmeal made with raisins and low-fat milk
- Strawberry smoothie made with low-fat milk

Midmorning Snack

Small, intermittent meals keep your metabolism working.

- Piece of fruit
- Whole grain toast with almond butter spread
- Graham cracker with peanut butter and low-fat chocolate milk

Lunch

Remember to eat smaller, more consistent meals.

- Bowl of mixed fresh fruits; whole grain toast topped by carrot salad and tuna
- Chicken wrap with lettuce and hummus
- Green salad with hard-boiled eggs and carrots
- Tuna salad on rice crackers; sliced apples
- Whole wheat tortilla with avocado and tomato
- Whole wheat pita sandwich with turkey and vegetables; pretzels; low-fat milk
- Rice bowl with beans, cheese, salsa, and avocado; whole grain tortilla chips
- Low-fat tuna-melt sandwich; fruit cup; low-fat yogurt

Midafternoon Snack

Keep all snacks low in sugar.

- Apple chips
- Fat-free yogurt
- Berry smoothie with non-fat yogurt

Dinner

In the spirit of several small meals spread throughout the day, dinner should not be a time for super-sizing portions.

- White bean stew; slice of whole grain bread
- Baked salmon; sweet potatoes; green beans
- Vegetable salad; grilled chicken
- Tomatoes stuffed with rice
- Stir-fried vegetables and tofu; brown rice
- Grilled papaya chicken; brown rice

Evening Snack

The anti-oxidants in both of these make them a perfect treat.

- Small piece of chocolate (70 percent cocoa)
- Glass of red wine

THE VEGETARIAN EXERCISER

If you are a vegetarian, you can still exercise with energy. It is true that a vegetarian diet generally has a lower protein intake (because humans digest plant protein less easily than animal protein). Vegetarian athletes should be sure to get 1.3–1.8 grams of plant protein daily for each kilogram of body weight.

D. Enette Larson-Meyer, a licensed dietitian and member of the Academy of Nutrition and Dietetics, suggests that vegetarian athletes can easily take in sufficient protein, providing their diet is adequate in energy sources and contains a variety of plant-protein foods, such as legumes, grains, nuts, and seeds. For example, a male athlete weighing 176 pounds (80 kilograms) and consuming 3,600 calories would receive 1.41 grams of protein per kilogram of body weight from the average vegetarian diet and 1.2 grams of protein per kilogram of body weight from the average vegan diet. (A vegan diet contains no animal-derived protein sources. For example, vegans do not eat meat, fish, eggs, or dairy foods.) A 110-pound (50-kilogram) female athlete consuming 2,200 calories per day would receive 1.38 grams of protein per kilogram of body weight from a vegetarian diet and 1.21 grams of protein per kilogram of body weight from a vegan diet. Therefore, most vegetarian athletes meet the requirements for endurance training without special meal planning. Strength-trained athletes (weight lifters, wrestlers, football players, or field throwers), or those with high training levels or low energy intakes, may need to include more protein-rich foods. This is easily accomplished, Larson-Meyer says, by encouraging the athletes to add one to three servings of protein-rich foods to their current diet (e.g., a soy milk shake, lentils with spaghetti sauce, tofu added to a stir-fry, or garbanzo beans added to a salad).

If you are a vegetarian, be aware that you may be at risk for low levels of Vitamin B12, Vitamin D, riboflavin, iron, calcium, and zinc.

- ***Vitamin B12***. Your vegetarian diet can provide you with most of the required B vitamins. Vitamin B12, however, may be the exception, depending on your diet. Due to the vitamin's function in maintaining the blood and nervous systems, its effect on vegetarian athletic performance has been studied. In fact, injections of Vitamin B12 are still used by some athletes/coaches because of the belief that oxygen delivery is increased (which in turn enhances endurance). Since cobalamin, the active form of Vitamin B12, is found exclusively in animal products, vegan athletes need to regularly consume B12-fortified foods, which include nutritional yeast and fortified brands of soy milk, breakfast cereals, and meat analogs. Vegetarians who consume eggs, cheese, milk, and yogurt receive an ample supply of this vitamin.

- ***Riboflavin***. Several studies have suggested that riboflavin needs may be increased in some vegetarians who begin an exercise program. Be particularly aware of this if you are starting with a marginal riboflavin status. Since riboflavin intakes are reportedly low in some vegans, you should learn the plant sources of riboflavin to ensure adequate intake. These include avocados, nuts, sea vegetables, soybeans, dark green leafy vegetables, and whole grain cereals.

- ***Antioxidant vitamins***. Vitamins C and E may protect you against exercise-induced "oxidative stress." Several recent reviews have summarized the current understanding: Antioxidant supplements are potentially beneficial in protecting against free radical production and oxidation of fat, but supplements have not been shown to enhance exercise performance. As a vegetarian athlete, you may have an advantage over your meat-eating counterparts, since antioxidants are readily obtained from a diet rich in nuts, seeds, vegetables, and vegetable oils.

- ***Vitamin D***. Vitamin D is essential for bone formation and the absorption of calcium and phosphorus. It is present in oily fish, eggs, and dairy products but not in plant foods. Vegans can obtain Vitamin D from vegetable margarines, some soy milks, and foods that are fortified with the vitamin. It is also manufactured by your skin when you are exposed to sunlight, so you can usually get enough Vitamin D this way to meet your body's requirements; eating fortified foods ensures that you get adequate amounts as an athlete. Some vegans may need a Vitamin D supplement.

- ***Iron***. All athletes are at risk of iron depletion and iron deficiency anemia. However, iron loss is increased in some athletes, particularly rigorously training female endurance athletes, due to gastrointestinal bleeding, heavy sweating, and hemolysis (the destruction of red blood cells, caused by disruption of the cell membrane and resulting in the release of hemoglobin). Hemolysis is seen in some types of anemia, which can be either inherited or acquired, for example, by exposure to toxins or by the presence of antibodies that attack red blood cells. Insufficient iron intake or reduced absorption, however, are the most probable causes of poor iron status. Some studies have found female vegetarian runners have a similar iron intake but a lower iron status than non-vegetarian runners. As a vegetarian, you do not absorb iron as readily as you would if you consumed meat. Your endurance may be affected, even without anemia, if you have low iron stores.

In most cases, vegetarian athletes can achieve proper iron status without iron supplementation, according to the Vegetarian Nutrition Dietetics Practice Group of the Academy of Nutrition and Dietetics. However, as a vegetarian, you need to be knowledgeable about plant sources of iron and factors that enhance and interfere with iron absorption. For example, if you consume milk or tea with beans at lunch, you may have to replace the beverage with citrus juice to enhance iron absorption at that meal. In some cases, vegetarian athletes may temporarily require supplements to build up or maintain iron stores. You should have your iron status monitored if you are taking an iron supplement because there could be side effects.

- ***Calcium***. Low calcium intake has been associated with an increased risk of stress fractures and low bone density, particularly in female athletes who are not menstruating. The major source of calcium in Western diets is generally milk and dairy products. If you are a vegan, you can obtain enough calcium from plant foods. Good sources include dried fruits, nuts, seeds, tofu, leafy green vegetables, and watercress. Also, white bread is fortified with calcium, as are some soy milks. Hard water can also provide significant amounts of calcium. Recommendations for active vegetarian men and premenopausal women is the same as the RDA, which is 800 milligrams for adults. Calcium intake, however, is one of many factors associated with calcium balance and accounts for only 11 percent of its variation. Urinary calcium excretion, on the other hand, accounts for 51 percent of the variation in calcium balance and is influenced by dietary protein, sodium, and possibly phosphoric acid. Vegans (and possibly vegetarians who consume few dairy products) may have lower calcium requirements because of their lower intakes of animal protein, total protein, and sodium, which increase kidney calcium excretion. However, until more is known about calcium requirements for vegetarians, you would be wise to meet the RDA for calcium.

- ***Zinc.*** Although little is known regarding the zinc status of vegetarian athletes, some dieticians think vegetarians may not have sufficient absorption of zinc from plant foods because plants are lower in zinc than animal products. You can obtain zinc from fortified cereals, hard cheeses, legumes, nuts, miso, tofu, wheat germ, and whole grain products.

HOME**WORK**

If you are what you eat, let's find out what you're made of. Start the following three good habits today:

1. Begin a food diary that lists everything you put in your mouth, including how much and at what time.
2. Review your list periodically to determine the food items that you most regularly consume—and determine whether they are smart choices.
3. Make one positive food pattern change. (Perhaps, like me, you may choose to stop consuming sugar and improve your life!)

"Success is the sum of small efforts—
repeated day in and day out."

—Robert Collier, author of
The Law of the Higher Potential

CHAPTER **FOURTEEN**

14

"In the Mouth of the Wolf"—Creating Your Mental Edge

"In bocca al lupo . . . in bocca al lupo. . . . Crepe lupo!" This Italian expression is the mantra I repeat over and over at the end of a long (or faster-than-usual) race to keep myself going. It is the mental edge of my game.

We all need a mantra to keep us going—especially when our bodies have taken up camp with the enemy. That mental edge is important because, at some point, it is all in your head—whether you are simply trying to motivate yourself to step away from the couch each day, or to run to the next light pole before you stop to walk, or (when you are at the end of a long, hard race and need to "twist the towel," if you will) to get the last drops of energy out of your body.

So here I am at mile 20 of a marathon—6.2 miles to go, and I began feeling tired at mile 18. By mile 20, my legs are still my allies, but my core and buttocks are screaming, since I am a typical runner and don't spend enough time working on them. The streets are filled with well-meaning fans waving, cheering, and yelling "you are almost there"—but 6.2 miles is *not* almost there. *In bocca al lupo* means "in the mouth of the wolf." I feel like I am in the mouth of the wolf, facing down this physical and mental challenge I am 20 miles into. I hear the muffled sound of the crowd around me, but I am all in my head and I hear myself talking. This race is bigger than this moment. I've been training daily for six months, and yet it is all about this moment. So I repeat: *"In bocca al lupo . . . in bocca al lupo."* And my triumphant response is: *"Crepe lupo!"* Slay the wolf! I will not be overtaken in this moment, and I keep running.

Believe it or not, I borrowed this Italian expression from several of my opera singer friends. It is their version of "break a leg." Imagine you are one voice about to take the stage where you will battle, without microphones, to not only be heard but brilliantly heard as you vie to resonate over the voices of an 80-piece orchestra, 30 chorus members, and several other principal singers before more than 2,000 people in the hall. The opera singer stands in the wings of the stage, viewing her playing field. If she fails, it is a public failure, known in the hall, in the newspapers, and around the world. She is looking into the mouth of the wolf. *"In bocca al lupo,"* one singer says to another. *"Crepe lupo!"* is the firm reply, as defeat is *not* an option.

Choosing a mantra, a word, a phrase, a name, or a song that means "I will not be defeated in this moment" is one important part of mental training.

WHAT IS MENTAL TRAINING?

Mental training, also known as sport psychology or performance enhancement, is similar to physical skills training in that the goal is to prepare athletes to consistently perform their best. While physical training focuses on teaching your body proper execution of skills, mental training focuses on teaching your mind to remove mental barriers that might hinder your performance. Mental training is an individualized program that teaches you how to identify and re-create your ideal mindset in order to perform your best in competition and in practice. Mental training gives athletes the knowledge and ability to control their thinking, their emotions, and, in turn, their performance. Teams can benefit from mental training as well. Mental training gives the individual athlete and teams the competitive edge they need to take their game to a higher level.

DISPELLING SOME MENTAL TRAINING MYTHS

Many athletes and coaches claim that at least 60 percent of their sport is mental; however, most people spend little if any time working on the mental aspects of their sport. Coaches say one reason for this is that there is not enough time for physical training, let alone mental training. However, while the schedules of coaches and athletes are limited, mental training does not require a lot of extra time after the initial learning stage. In fact, mental training is most effective when it can be incorporated into everyday practice and competition, enhancing the quality of both.

Another reason coaches and athletes give for not working on their mental game is that mental training is only for elite athletes. While it is true that many of the top athletes in the world do engage in mental training, athletes of all ages and levels can benefit from enhancing their abilities to control their minds. Whether they are building confidence, increasing concentration, or controlling their anxiety, athletes of all ages and abilities can use a variety of mental training techniques both in sport and in life.

Another common myth is that mental training is only for athletes with problems. On the contrary, mental training is most effective when it is used to *prevent* performance problems from occurring rather than to provide a quick fix to a performance slump.

HOW DO YOU RAISE THE BAR?

As you are thinking about your own mental edge, work through the following mental training skills.

Consistently Perform at Your Peak

- Ask yourself what you can do to make today better than yesterday. Work on this.
- Don't settle for being comfortable. Striving for more enhances performance.
- Don't settle for what's "good enough for today." Go above and beyond the minimum expected of you.

Know What Drives You and Stay Focused on These Motivators

- How do you define excellence?
- What are you trying to accomplish?
- What drives you to be better?
- What do you like about what you are doing?
- What is your view of yourself?

Set Goals for Success

- Don't just set out to "try your hardest." Set specific goals so you can measure whether or not you accomplished them.
- Make sure your goals are challenging but realistic and know when you want to accomplish them.
- Focus small, don't get ahead of yourself, and take it one thing at a time.
- Focus on process goals (the fundamentals you need to perform well), not only on outcome goals.
- Set goals for every aspect of your life.

- Keep goals positive.
- Set up a support system, tell people your goals, and ask them to reinforce your efforts.
- Write your goals down. This is very important!

Know the Types of Goals

- Realize that on a day-to-day basis, you will see the most improvement by focusing on the fundamentals that are necessary to succeed, not on the final results you want to achieve. Thus, setting goals is extremely important in helping you to reach your peak. There are three sets of goals you need to know about:
    1. *Outcome goals* focus on the results (winning, being the best). This type of goal is motivating but usually outside your immediate control.
    2. *Performance goals* focus on improvements relative to your own past performance (e.g., time improvement).
    3. *Process goals* are related to procedures engaged in during performance (workout plan, stride, focus). You totally control process goals and the focus is on self-improvement, so they keep you motivated in the face of obstacles.

Use Your Goals to Motivate You

- Focus on and reward your process goals.
- Develop goal buddies.
- Establish daily reminders (for instance, you can use a motto).
- Establish goal-focused workouts (workout plans that move toward your overall goal).

- Picture your desired achievements.
- Have a weekly theme.

Develop the Midas Touch

- Don't sell yourself short. Make today your day.
- Ask yourself: "What can I improve upon today?"
- Focus on what you want to accomplish in every situation.
- Know what you are working toward.

MORE THAN JUST PERFORMANCE

While mental training is most commonly used to help individual or team performance, several other issues can be addressed through mental training. First, mental training can assist athletes who are injured in dealing with stress, in expediting the rehabilitation process, and in mentally preparing to return to competition. Second, a mental training consultant can help to educate parents and coaches on ways to enhance a young athlete's sport experience. Talking with groups about their influence on athletes' lives not only helps to ensure a positive sport experience for the athletes but also assists in opening the lines of communication among parents, coaches, and athletes. Third, mental training can assist athletes outside of sport in developing life skills, working through major life decisions, and transitioning out of sport.

As you proceed toward the remainder of this book, equipped to take control and age in the best possible way through exercise, look into the mouth of your wolf and F.A.C.E. your future without fear. *Crepe lupo!*

HOMEWORK

Do you have a mantra to keep you going? If not, Google inspirational quotes and choose one that really moves you.

Now set a goal, and fill out the following lines:

- My long-term goal is: ______________________________

  ____

  ____

- My goal for this week is: ______________________________

  ____

  ____

- What can I do to achieve this? ______________________________

  ____

  ____

- What obstacles might I face, and how can I overcome them? _____

  ____

  ____

- What will result from my achieving this goal? ______________

  ____

  ____

Make a statement.

- My mission this year is to: ______________________________

  ____

  ____

- Every day I will: ______________________________

  ____

  ____

"I think it's quite great to set yourself a big challenge, and then you've got another reason for keeping fit."

—Sir Richard Branson, inventor, entrepreneur, and visionary

CHAPTER FIFTEEN

15

When the Shoe Fits, Wear It

At this point, you have so much inspiration that you are probably raring to go, and if you are, then just go right now before the surge of energy passes. I hope you have been flexing, walking, resisting, and balancing as you prepared yourself through this book. One additional bit of preparation not to be overlooked is your equipment. (I don't want you to add "I have nothing to wear" to the list of excuses that can crop up for not working out!) Even the best training can get sidetracked if your shoes rub blisters on your feet, your clothes don't wick moisture, or your equipment fails. Preparation makes perfect performance.

LETTER FROM A LONGTIME MASTERS ATHLETE

I have run many races with my 75-year-old father, Gene Wright. I am always fascinated and amused to watch how deliberately he addresses his equipment before a race. When writing this book, I decided to get his take on how he chooses footwear and ask him to dispense advice about how you might organize yourself for fitness after 40 and prepare yourself for a road race. He responded in the form of a letter to you:

Hello, fitness after 40 enthusiasts:

Welcome to a great life. Now that you have made the decision to take control of the quality of your life and the aging process, I would like to give you a few thoughts and hints about the equipment you need.

Beginning to exercise on a consistent basis requires very little equipment. And what you *do* need is inexpensive and readily available. You probably have most of it in your dresser already. The hard-and-fast rule concerning equipment is that it must be comfortable. If any part of your equipment is uncomfortable when you put it on, it will get really uncomfortable when you are exercising in it.

What do you need? The first (and most important) thing is a pair of shoes. The decisions you make concerning what brand and what type of shoes to buy should take some time and effort. When you buy your shoes, I suggest that you go to a salesperson who is knowledgeable about shoes.

Your shoes should be specific to your sport. There are walking shoes, running shoes, tennis shoes, and good old sneakers for tooling around the house. Know what you need. If you are walking, you can get away with a pair of running shoes, but not the reverse. (Walking shoes are usually too stiff for running.) If you are in the market for a pair of running shoes, go to a shop that specializes in running shoes and has staff that actually run. They will analyze the shoe's fit on your foot and talk to you about what kind of workout you do. If you don't know where to find a running shoe store, go to www.runnersworld.com and hit the bar for "Shoes and Gear." (When you get to that page, you will see a section called "Tools," and there, an icon for "Store Finder." When you go to that section, you will find stores listed by state.)

Remember the following when you are at the store: Your shoes should caress your feet. (Examine the cushioning and support.) Typically, your athletic shoes should be one to two sizes larger than your street shoes. You need more room in the toe and mid-foot areas; these shoes are just built that way. You also need more room because during exercise, your feet get bigger and they need room to expand. You also do not want to inhibit the circulation in your feet. In addition, you probably do not want the most expensive shoe you can get, and you certainly do not want the cheapest shoe on the market. A midpriced shoe is often best. You can usually get a pair for $80 to $100.

Take your time in the shoe store because this piece of equipment can make or break your workout. If you have a pair of shoes that you walk or run in already, it is best to bring them with you so the staff can look at the tread and how you wear out your shoes. If you wear inserts, bring them, too, since the staff can use all this information to help you choose the best shoe for your foot. Also, make sure you take the socks you are going to wear while exercising. You want to guarantee a perfect fit.

Very quickly, there will be several pairs of shoes around you on the floor, and probably two or three pairs that you have decided you might want. Try the first pair on. How do the shoes feel? Walk around in them. If the store has a treadmill, walk a few minutes on it while wearing the shoes. If you feel any rough spot, tight area, or discomfort, take them off and try the next pair. If the shoes are too tight, you will end up pounding your big toenails and losing them, rubbing your skin raw, compressing the nerves that wrap around your sole, or having numb toes. Keep trying on different pairs until your feet are caressed and you are completely happy with the shoes.

In short, be very particular when you are buying your shoes. They are the foundation of all that you do. If your feet are not comfortable, all other parts of your body will be affected. The wrong shoes may cause discomfort and injuries. If you have purchased a pair of shoes that you like, stick with them.

My best advice is to be deliberate, take your time, and don't skimp on your shoes.

See you on the road,

Gene Wright

GETTING THE BASICS

Believe it or not, to get started, shoes (and a good sports bra, if you're a woman) are all you really need. For your first foray off the couch, you can throw on whatever cotton T-shirt you have in the back of your drawer. Don't let "getting the perfect gear" slow down your process of getting started. My advice: Get your shoes—and get going!

Shoes

To get started, you may be tempted to grab that old, shriveled-up pair of workout shoes that have been lying around in the back of your closet since the 1980s. This is *not* the way to put your best foot forward. Of all the possible new "gear" you could buy, the one piece you truly can't move without is a well-fitting pair of shoes. The right shoes can make or break your workout, so it's important to get it right. The best way to get the right footwear is to shop at a specialty shoe store instead of a department store.

Only wear the shoes that fit.

Our feet change considerably as we age, and for women, as we have children. They get both longer and wider. Go to a reputable sports equipment store and let the clerk measure both of your feet while you are standing. You may be surprised at your new size.

Many exercise shoes come in multiple widths per length. Aging causes the most problems with the front of the foot (forefoot), including pain (metatarsalgia) and bunions. This makes the width and height of the front of the shoe key. Even if the clerk measures your foot and brings out that size, the shoes may not fit correctly, so experiment until you find a pair that does. Shoe sizing varies per company. If your feet measured different sizes, begin trying on the bigger size.

Make sure you choose the type of shoe made for the activity you are doing. For instance, running shoes have little to no lateral support, since running is a forward-backward (not side-to-side) sport. For the best running shoe fit, stand in your new shoes, wiggle your toes, and measure the distance between your longest toe and the end of the shoe. It should equal the width of your thumb.

If you are cross-training, playing tennis or basketball or any sport with side-to-side movement, you should choose a shoe with lateral support. The shoe should be more true to your foot size than a running shoe, but still neither cramp your foot nor allow it to slide. Cross-trainers, for walking, need a good heel and midfoot support (you will not be able to bend the shoe easily); these are also lightweight.

Athletic shoes are designed with different foot types in mind. In general, there are three foot types: normal, flat (pronated), and high-arched (supinated). Each type has different issues. To determine which type you are, take the "wet test." With a damp foot, step onto a piece of colored paper or cardboard. If your footprint looks like a regular foot, you probably have normal feet. If your footprint looks almost rectangular, you have flat feet. If you see only the ball, toes, and heel with little in between, you have high-arched feet.

If you have normal feet, you have minimal calluses and can wear any shoe with moderate support. By comparison, if you have flat feet, they roll in excessively. This can cause calluses, bunions, neuromas (masses surrounding nerves between your toes), plantar fasciitis, and stress fractures of the bones in the forefoot. Flat feet require maximum support with motion-control shoes and firm midsoles. This means that the shoes have strong plastic heel counters, firm plastic inserts in the midfoot portion, and a wider stable base of support. Flat feet do not need highly cushioned shoes. Flat-footed exercisers should look for labels that say "motion control." This means that the shoe is stiffer and does part of the job your foot should do to stay stable.

On the other hand, a high-arched foot has poor shock absorption. This leads to more ankle sprains, pain under the big toe (sesamoiditis), calluses, and hammertoes (where the second through fifth toes bend up and hit the top of the shoe). High-arched feet need shoes that allow plenty of motion and have cushion. People with high-arched feet should look for labels that say "absorb," "gel," "air," and "hydroflow."

When you think you have found the right type and size of shoe, do a test jog around the store or on the treadmill most stores have for this purpose. Make sure you still have the same good fit you felt standing when you are in motion. Uncomfortable cramping or sliding around in the shoe will rapidly become pain during a workout. Finally, try balancing on one foot. Your foot should fit centered over the sole of the shoe and should not spill out around the sides.

Love your shoes when you get them home—but not too much.

After completing your workout and activity, take the shoes off. Your workout shoes should not be your shoes for running around town doing a thousand errands. This will cause early breakdown and even aches and pains during workouts. For running round town, get some comfy shoes that look good and put your workout shoes away.

Another mistake we make with our workout shoes is loving them for years . . . and years . . . and years. If you are a runner or walker, replace your shoes every 300 to 500 miles. If you are not a runner, then once a year is usually good.

When I really love my running shoes but they reach their limit, I stop running in them but keep them around for dog walks, yard work, or errands. That way, I can still love them, just not too much.

Support on Top

For women, I have one more key suggestion: a great-fitting sports bra. There are many different types today, and just like you do with your everyday bras, you should try them on and consider several features. A sports bra should not simply smash your breasts against your body. It must support your figure.

While in the store, jump up and down, jog in place, and raise and lower your arms. How does it feel? Are you still inside it? Is it comfortable? Does it dig into your skin or bind you up? Finally, fabric is important. Cotton generally stays wet and cold, so look at the new synthetic blends. Many high-tech fabrics are capable of wicking moisture away from your body so that it evaporates.

Little Extras Make All the Difference

Let me tell you, sweat on raw skin hurts, so don't forget body lubricant. Silicone-based ointment works nicely to prevent chafing under the arms, between the thighs, or anywhere that rubs.

As you get serious about your new routine, you'll want to choose comfortable, slimming workout clothes that are not baggy. Clothes that are too loose, too short, or too tight make using gym machines or getting on the floor difficult. Also, don't overdress. If you stay cool, you are more likely to continue exercising. Again, when you are buying these clothes, make sure no areas rub or chafe your skin.

You can add gadgets and gear—such as wicking fabric, heart rate and distance monitors, compression wear, and so forth—after you get through the first few weeks of working out. You could even make a new piece of fancy, high-tech equipment your reward after you complete the Six-Week Jump Start to Mobility Plan that we discussed in Chapter 10. Set your sights on it now and work toward your reward as you change your life.

GETTING YOUR MOVE ON

You do not need a gym to work out. Any space and your own weights will do. Sometimes, however, it is easier to stay motivated if you have a place to go and a variety of activities to do. I encourage my patients to join a gym for just this reason. For some, affording the membership is an issue. My answer to this excuse is to turn your cable off and invest the money in a gym membership. In addition, today, there are many gym specials and you can shop around for the best deal.

Choosing a Gym

In order to get the most from your money, here are a few tips on choosing the best gym.

- ***Location, location, location***. It doesn't matter if you are thinking about joining the Taj Mahal of gyms; if it is not easily accessible to you, you will not go frequently. You think you will now, when you are romanced by the gym's bells and whistles, but you won't. Choose a gym that is less than 10 minutes from your home or work and that has easy access to parking, if you drive.

- ***Activities, toys, and equipment***. Think about how you like to exercise. Are you a class joiner, a spinner, a runner, a lap swimmer? Do you like Pilates, yoga, aerobics? Your gym should have a wide variety of activities that you like to do. It must also have floor space for stretching with an abundance of exercise toys, such as exercise balls, stools, and rubber tubing. It should have both machine and free weights. Does the gym have adequate numbers of solo cardio machines and weight equipment to ensure that you won't wait forever? Does the equipment accommodate all skill levels and sizes?

- ***Environment and condition***. Is the aerobics floor wooden or suspended? (Both are easier on the joints than concrete.) What is the condition of the equipment? Is it clean? Run your finger along the equipment. If it is dirty or sticky, beware. Are there bottles of disinfectant near the equipment groups? You want a gym that expects members to towel off the equipment with disinfectant after they use it. Alternatively, there should be an attendant who does this after every client. Look down at the carpet and at the showers. Are they clean?

- ***Trial pass***. Most gyms give potential members weekly passes to try the place out. Visit during a time you are likely to work out. When you visit, look around at whom you will be exercising with. Do you feel comfortable? Is staff available to answer your questions or assist you? If the idea of working out among professional hard bodies makes you feel shy, you might try your local YMCA, community center, or college athletic center instead. For women who are uncomfortable working out around men, choose a gym that allows only women or has designated women-only areas. Does the gym offer fitness testing and program orientation?

- ***Hours***. While most gyms are not open 24/7, they must be open early and stay open late to accommodate you. This includes weekends.

- ***Fees***. Gyms usually charge an initiation fee and a monthly fee. Does the monthly fee include everything, or will you pay extra for the "good stuff" or to be there during prime time? Can you bring a guest, and if so, how often and for what fee?

- ***Staff***. Besides having a good attitude, the staff at a gym should be trained in both first aid and CPR. They should also be certified by an organization such as the American Council on Exercise (ACE), the American College of Sports Medicine (ACSM), or the National Academy of Sports Medicine (NASM).

Considering Your Personal Trainer

Sometimes we all need a helping hand, and a personal trainer can be just the right addition to your fitness plan. A personal trainer can assist you in evaluating your fitness level, planning a program, and keeping you motivated. Sometimes you need someone standing over your shoulder to push yourself to the next level. In addition, a personal trainer should be able to educate you about F.A.C.E.-ing your future.

You must be careful, however, to choose a trainer who understands what *you* want to accomplish and the unique qualities of the mature athlete and active ager. The trainer must understand that you are not merely a bad sequel to your 20-year-old self but are, in fact, unique. I recommend finding a trainer who has previously worked with masters athletes and adult-onset exercisers. Interview trainers to find out if they believe that fitness after 40 is possible. Although many great therapists and trainers are out there, you would be surprised by how many of them buy into the notion that we should all just slow down when we reach a certain arbitrary age. Such a belief will affect how a trainer would work with you.

Just like any service, one great way to find a personal trainer is to ask your friends, family, business associates, and so forth if they are working with anyone they like. You can also watch the personal trainers who work at your gym and observe how they work with people. If you see trainers you like, ask to talk to them about your goals. You also want to choose a personal trainer who is certified. You can find a list of certified personal trainers online at certification.acsm.org/pro-finder, www.nsca.org, or acefitness.org/acefit/locate-trainer.

If you decide to hire a personal trainer, do so for a short period of time first. Then, if you are achieving your goals, you can purchase additional sessions. It would be unfortunate to buy a six-month package of training sessions only to find out you don't get along with the trainer or she doesn't understand your goals.

The International Council on Active Aging (ICAA) has put together a great guide for choosing a personal fitness trainer qualified to work with you. (Look for it on their website at www.icaa.cc/consumer/welcomeback/personaltrainerguide.pdf.) It consists of specific questions you can use to interview your potential trainer and the responses you are looking for.

Here is a list of general areas to consider:

- ***Education***. Your trainer must be certified by the American College of Sports Medicine, American Council on Exercise, or the National Strength and Conditioning Association. Ideally, he would also have a degree in exercise science or a related college degree.
- ***Experience***. Although everyone has to start somewhere, try to choose a trainer who has several years of experience in an area related to your specific goals. Regardless of whether you are a cyclist, a runner, a swimmer, or do something else entirely, you want someone who understands your sport. Also, if you have specific medical conditions, you want a trainer who has had experience with other people with these conditions. Does the trainer have experience helping people in your age group maximize their performance? Does the trainer understand the strategies for injury prevention in the masters athlete?
- ***Personality and professionalism***. You will be working closely with your personal trainer, so does she seem like a person whose personality meshes with yours? Does she listen to you and what your goals are, or do you sense that she has her

own agenda? Does she keep up with the latest technology? What does she expect of you?

- ***Logistics***. Does this trainer come to your particular gym, and will he come to your home or local park? What hours is he available? How does he prefer to be paid? Does he have liability insurance?
- ***Trial run***. Before committing to a package of training sessions, take a trial run. Evaluate how you feel working with this person. Does she listen to you? Are the workouts varied and in line with what you have read in this book? Did she give you hints about form and lifestyle as you worked out?

HOME**WORK**

If you decide to hire a personal trainer, you must first interview the people you are considering. Do not be afraid to ask the questions outlined above. Remember that you are entrusting your body to this person and you want to make sure you are the focus of the trainer's interest. You can help your trainer to help you by putting some thought into what kind of fitness goals you want to achieve. As discussed in Chapter 14, setting and writing down goals makes it easier to achieve them. Be able to tell your trainer the answers to the following questions:

- *Specifically, what do you want to achieve by hiring him?* For instance, you could say: "I want to lose five pounds in the next five weeks," "I want to be supervised while I work through the four components of F.A.C.E.-ing my future," "I want to work up to walking three miles," or "I want to evaluate my muscle weaknesses and focus on strengthening them."

- *Exactly what do you want your body to look like?* If you see a picture of the kind of legs, abdomen, or arms you would like to have, bring the picture to show her.
- *How much time will you commit to achieving these goals?* For instance: "I can meet with you for one hour four times a week, and one session must be on a Saturday."
- *How do you like to learn?* Do you like a lot of demonstration or coaching? Think also about how you are motivated. Do you respond to coaching that is more encouraging (for instance, "Great job, that was fantastic form. In the next set, let's turn it up a notch")? Or do you prefer coaching that is more critical in style (for instance, "Your form was off, focus on the next set")? This is important. If criticism does not motivate you, you will resent your trainer using this method and you will not progress as well as if he used a more encouraging style. The reverse is also true.

A Closing Word on *Your* Fitness After 40

Despite the common dogma that life slides over the hill at some arbitrary age, I hope by now you love these middle years as much as I do! My ability to make choices that control my body, brains, and bliss (from what I see in the mirror down to the tiniest stem cell inside) is an amazing and hopeful position to be in—and I love it. I truly believe that these can be the best years of your life, too. Now that you know that *you* control your trajectory of health and aging, I hope you share my excitement and are ready to F.A.C.E. your future of fitness after 40!

I would love to hear about your journey and triumphs! Connect with me via my website www.drvondawright.com or via Facebook.com/DrVonda and Twitter @DrVondaWright.

FURTHER RESOURCES

DR. WRIGHT'S FAVORITE ONLINE SITES

I am beginning this section with a list of my favorite online sites. The Internet holds a bounty of information on fitness. Whether you are looking for instruction, scientific articles, or a source of equipment (or you simply want to have a talk with other active agers), there is a site for you. Here are a few of the sites that I especially like:

- www.drvondawright.com: My professional website, blog, and sources of generally great things for fitness after 40
- www.womenshealthconversations.com: Women's Health Conversations, a live conference series and online resource to educate and empower smart, savvy women to make the best health choices for themselves and everyone they touch
- www.aaos.org: American Academy of Orthopaedic Surgeons
- www.sportsmed.org: American Orthopaedic Society for Sports Medicine

- www.icaa.cc: International Council on Active Aging
- www.nsga.com: National Senior Games Association
- www.sharecare.com: An amazing curated website connecting real patients and their questions to real medical experts and professional associations
- www.realage.com: There is a difference between your chronological age and your body's physiologic age (or your "RealAge") based on the lifestyle choices you make; check this out to determine how your lifestyle choices are affecting your longevity
- www.acefitness.org: American Council on Exercise, a reputable source of sports training information and a certifying agency for personal trainers

HELPFUL ORGANIZATIONS AND PUBLICATIONS

Academy of Nutrition and Dietetics (AND)
120 South Riverside Plaza, Suite 2000
Chicago, IL 60606
312-899-0040, 800-877-1600
www.eatright.org

The website of the Academy of Nutrition and Dietetics features comprehensive nutrition information for the public, including a database of dieticians in your area.

American Academy of Orthopaedic Surgeons (AAOS)
9400 West Higgins Road
Rosemont, IL 60018
847-823-7186; fax 847-823-8125
www.aaos.org

The American Academy of Orthopaedic Surgeons provides education and practice management services for orthopaedic surgeons and allied health professionals. It also serves as an advocate for improved patient care and informs the public about the science of orthopaedics.

American College of Sports Medicine (ACSM)
401 West Michigan Street
Indianapolis, IN 46202
317-637-9200; fax 317-634-7817
www.acsm.org

The ACSM is a national organization of physical therapists, exercise physiologists, athletic trainers, and fitness professionals. They provide guidance for all aspects of fitness and sports health, set standards for exercise prescription, and certify personal trainers.

American Council on Exercise (ACE)
4851 Paramount Drive
San Diego, CA 92123
858-576-6500, 888-825-3636; fax 858-576-6564
www.acefitness.org

The American Council on Exercise provides a search engine on its website that can help you locate a certified exercise professional in your area. ACE is the largest sports medicine and exercise science organization in the world. Nearly 50,000 members throughout the United States and the world are dedicated to promoting and integrating scientific research, education, and practical applications of sports medicine and exercise science to maintain and enhance physical performance, fitness, health, and quality of life.

American Medical Society for Sports Medicine (AMSSM)
4000 West 114th Street, Suite 100
Leawood, KS 66211

913-327-1415; fax 913-327-1491
www.amssm.org

The society fosters relationships among sports medicine specialists and provides educational resources for members, other sports medicine professionals, and the public.

American Orthopaedic Society for Sports Medicine (AOSSM)
9400 West Higgins Road, Suite 300
Rosemont, IL 60018
847-292-4900; fax 847-292-4905
www.sportsmed.org

The society is an organization of orthopaedic surgeons and allied health professionals dedicated to educating healthcare professionals and the public about sports medicine. It promotes and supports educational and research programs in sports medicine, including those concerned with fitness, as well as programs designed to advance knowledge of the recognition, treatment, rehabilitation, and prevention of athletic injuries.

American Physical Therapy Association (APTA)
1111 North Fairfax Street
Alexandria, VA 22314
703-684-2782, 800-999-2782; fax 703-684-7343
www.apta.org

The association is a national professional organization of physical therapists, physical therapist assistants, and physical therapy students. Its objectives are to improve physical therapy practice, research, and education to promote, restore, and maintain optimal physical function, wellness, fitness, and quality of life, especially as it relates to movement and health.

American Senior Fitness Association (ASFA)
P.O. Box 2575
New Smyrna Beach, FL 32170
386-423-6634, 888-689-6791; fax 877-365-3048
www.seniorfitness.net

The ASFA is a good resource for personal trainers and physical therapists to gain information and training for working with seniors. They publish an online newsletter called *Experience!* that summarizes the latest training techniques and research.

Arthritis Foundation
1330 West Peachtree Street, Suite 100
Atlanta, GA 30309
404-872-7100
www.arthritis.org

The mission of the Arthritis Foundation is to improve lives through the prevention, control, and cure of arthritis and related diseases by providing grants to researchers to help find a cure, prevention, or better treatment for arthritis. The website provides links to information about different conditions, treatments, community groups, and more.

International Coalition for Aging and Physical Activity (ICAPA)
www.humankinetics.com/icapa

The mission of ICAPA is to promote physical activity, exercise science, and fitness in the health and well-being of older persons and to promote international initiatives in research, clinical practice, and public policy in the area of aging and physical activity. The coalition organizes a World Congress on Aging and Physical Activity approximately every four years.

International Council on Active Aging (ICAA)
3307 Trutch Street
Vancouver, BC, Canada V6L 2T3
604–734-4466, 866-335-9777; fax 604-708-4464
www.icaa.cc

The International Council on Active Aging is dedicated to changing the way people age by uniting professionals in the retirement, assisted living, fitness, rehabilitation, and wellness fields to dispel society's myths about aging. The council helps these professionals to empower aging baby boomers and older adults to improve their quality of life and maintain their dignity.

National Athletic Trainers' Association (NATA)
1620 Valwood Parkway, Suite 115
Carrollton, TX 75006
214-637-6282; fax 214-637-2206
www.nata.org

The association enhances the quality of healthcare for athletes and those engaged in physical activity. It also advances the profession of athletic training through education and research in the prevention, evaluation, management, and rehabilitation of injuries.

National Senior Games Association (NSGA)
P.O. Box 82059
Baton Rouge, LA 70884
225-766-6800; fax 225-766-9115
www.nsga.com

The association is a not-for-profit member of the United States Olympic Committee dedicated to motivating senior men and women to lead a healthy lifestyle through the senior games movement. The organization governs the National Summer Senior Games, the largest multi-sport event in the world for seniors, and other national senior athletic events.

It is also an umbrella for member state organizations across the United States that host State Senior Games or Senior Olympics.

Vegetarian Resource Group (VRG)
P.O. Box 1463
Baltimore, MD 21203
410-366-8343
www.vrg.org

The Vegetarian Resource Group is a nonprofit organization dedicated to educating the public on vegetarianism and related issues. It provides guidelines for all types and levels of vegetarian athletes.

Women's Sports Foundation
424 West 33rd Street, Suite 340
New York, NY 10001
646-845-0273; fax 212-967-2757
www.womenssportsfoundation.org

This is one of the most complete websites for female athletes, both rookies and seasoned veterans. It has resources to help you play at the top of your game, as well as descriptions of more than 100 sports and fitness activities.

SELECTED REFERENCES

American Cancer Society. "Exercise Can Improve Breast Cancer Survival," www.aahf.info/sec_news/section/bc_survival_081105.htm.

American College of Sports Medicine Position Stand. "The Recommended Quantity and Quality of Exercise for Developing and Maintaining Cardiorespiratory and Muscular Fitness and Flexibility in Healthy Adults." *Medicine & Science in Sports & Exercise* 31(6): 916–920 (1999).

Beim, Gloria, and Winter, Ruth. *The Female Athlete's Body Book: How to Prevent and Treat Sports Injuries in Women and Girls* (New York: McGraw-Hill, 2003).

Blumenthal, James A.; Smith, Patrick J.; and Hoffman, Benson M. "Opinion and Evidence: Is Exercise a Viable Treatment for Depression?" *ACSM's Health and Fitness Journal* 16(4): 14–21 (2012).

Brandy, W. D., and Irion, J. M. "The Effect of Time on Static Stretch on the Flexibility of the Hamstring Muscles." *Physical Therapy* 74(9): 845–850 (1994).

Brandy, W. D.; Irion, J. M.; and Briggler, M. "The Effect of Static Stretch and Dynamic Range of Motion Training on Flexibility for the Hamstring Muscles." *Journal of Orthopaedic & Sports Physical Therapy* 27(4): 295–300 (1998).

Campbell, W. W., and Geik, R. A. "Nutritional Considerations for the Older Athlete." *Nutrition* 20(7–8): 603–608 (2004).

Chen, A.; Mears, S. C.; and Hawkins, R. J. "Orthopaedic Care of the Aging Athlete." *Journal of the American Academy of Orthopaedic Surgeons* 13(6): 407–416 (2005).

Convertino, V. A., et al. "American College of Sports Medicine Position Stand: Exercise and Fluid Replacement." *Medicine & Science in Sports & Exercise* 28(1): i–vii (1996).

Erickson, Kirk I.; Prakash, Ruchika S.; Voss, Michelle W.; Chaddock, Laura; Hu, Liang; Morris, Katherine S.; White, Siobhan M.; Wójcicki, Thomas R.; McAuley, Edward; and Kramer, Arthur F. "Aerobic Fitness Is Associated with Hippocampal Volume in Elderly Humans." *Hippocampus* 19(10): 1030–1039 (2009).

Feland, J. Brent; Myrer, J. William; Schulthies, Shane S.; Fellingham, Gill W.; and Measom, Gary W. "The Effect of Duration of Stretching of the Hamstring Muscle Group for Increasing Range of Motion in People Aged 65 Years or Older." *Physical Therapy* 81: 1110–1117 (2001).

Ferreira, Gustavo Nunes Tasca, et al. "Gains in Flexibility Related to Measures of Muscular Performance: Impact of Flexibility on Muscular Performance." *Clinical Journal of Sport Medicine* 17(4): 276–281 (2007).

Fiatarone, Maria A.; Marks, Elizabeth C.; Ryan, Nancy D.; Meredith, Carol N.; Lipsitz, Lewis A.; and Evans, William J. "High-Intensity Strength Training in Nonagenarians: Effects on Skeletal Muscle." *JAMA* 263(22): 3029–3034 (1990).

Frontera, Walter R., et al. "Skeletal Muscle Fiber Quality in Older Men and Women." *American Journal of Physiology—Cell Physiology* 279(3): C611–C618 (2000).

Frontera, Walter R.; Hughes, Virginia A.; Lutz, Karyn J.; and Evans, William J. "A Cross-Sectional Study of Muscle Strength and Mass in 45- to 78-Year-Old Men and Women." *Journal of Applied Physiology* 71: 644–650 (1991).

Goodpaster, Bret H.; Carlson, Catherine L.; Visser, Marjolein; Kelley, David E.; et al. "The Attenuation of Skeletal Muscle and Strength in the Elderly: The Health ABC Study." *Journal of Applied Physiology* 90(6): 2157–2165 (2001).

Holmes, Michelle D.; Chen, Wendy Y.; Feskanich, Diane; Kroenke, Candyce H.; and Colditz, Graham A. "Physical Activity and Survival After Breast Cancer Diagnosis." *JAMA* 293(20): 2479–2486 (2005).

Kammerlander, Christian; Braito, M.; Kates, Stephen; Jeske, Hans-Christian; Roth, Tobias; et al. "The Epidemiology of Sports-Related Injuries in Older Adults: A Central European Epidemiologic Study." *Aging—Clinical and Experimental Research* 24(5): 448–454 (2012).

Katzel, Leslie I.; Sorkin, John D.; and Fleg, Jerome L. "A Comparison of Longitudinal Changes in Aerobic Fitness in Older Endurance Athletes and Sedentary Men." *Journal of the American Geriatrics Society* 49(12): 1657–1664 (2001).

Korhonen, Marko T., et al. "Aging, Muscle Fiber Type, and Contractile Function in Sprint-Trained Athletes." *Journal of Applied Physiology* 101(3): 906–917 (2006).

Lee, Duck-chul; Pate, Russell R.; Lavie, Carl J.; Sui, Xuemei; Church, Timothy S.; and Blair, Steven N. "Leisure-Time Running Reduces All-Cause and Cardiovascular Mortality Risk." *Journal of the American College of Cardiology* 64(5): 472–481 (2014).

Lepers, Romuald; Knechtle, Beat; and Stapley, Paul. "Trends in Triathlon Performance: Effects of Sex and Age." *Sports Medicine* 43(9): 851–863 (2013).

Maharam, L. G., et al. "Masters Athletes: Factors Affecting Performance." *Sports Medicine* 28(4): 273–285 (1999).

Maron, B. J., et al. "Recommendations for Preparticipation Screening and the Assessment of Cardiovascular Disease in Master Athletes." *Journal of the American Heart Association* 103(2): 327–334 (2001).

Meltzer, David E. "Body-Mass Dependence of Age-Related Deterioration in Human Muscular Function." *Journal of Applied Physiology* 80(4): 1149–1155 (1996).

Mosekilde, Lise. "Age-Related Changes in Bone Mass, Structure, and Strength—Effects of Loading." *Journal Zeitschrift für Rheumatologie* 59 (Suppl. 1): I1–I9 (2000); also *Rheumatol* 59(1): 1–9 (2000).

Pyron, Martha I. "The Aging Athlete: Risks and Benefits of Exercise." *Current Opinion in Orthopaedics* 13(2): 128–133 (2002).

Ribisl, Paul M. "Clinical Applications: Toxic 'Waist' Dump: Our Abdominal Visceral Fat." *ACSM's Health and Fitness Journal* 8(4): 22–25 (2004).

Rosenbloom, C. A., and Dunaway, A. "Nutrition Recommendations for Masters Athletes." *Clinics in Sports Medicine* 26(1): 91–100 (2007).

Shaw, Jonathan. "The Deadliest Sin: From Survival of the Fittest to Staying Fit Just to Survive: Scientists Probe the Benefits of Exercise—and the Dangers of Sloth." *Harvard Magazine* (March–April 2004).

Slentz, Cris Allan; Aiken, Lori B.; Houmard, Joseph A.; et al. "Inactivity, Exercise, and Visceral Fat. STRRIDE: A Randomized, Controlled Study of Exercise Intensity and Amount." *Journal of Applied Physiology* 99(4): 1613–1618 (2005).

Sowers, MaryFran R., et al. "Sarcopenia Is Related to Physical Functioning and Leg Strength in Middle-Aged Women." *Journals of Gerontology: Series A: Biological Sciences & Medical Sciences* 60: 486–490 (2005).

"Sports Injuries." U.S. Department of Health and Human Services, National Institutes of Health, National Institutes of Arthritis and Skin Diseases. NIH Publication No. 04–5278 (April 2004).

Tanaka, Hirofumi, and Seals, Douglas R. "Dynamic Exercise Performance in Masters Athletes: Insight into the Effects of Primary Human Aging on Physiological Functional Capacity." *Journal of Applied Physiology* 95(5): 2152–2162 (2003).

Taylor, Dean, et al. "Viscoelastic Properties of Muscle-Tendonitis: The Biomechanical Effects of Stretching." *American Journal of Sports Medicine* 18(3): 300–309 (1990).

UniSci. "Diet, Exercise Slow Prostate Cancer as Much as 30 Percent." www.unisci.com/stories/20013/0911013.htm.

"Visceral Fat Build-Up Is the High Cost of Inactivity." *Science Daily* (14 September 2005); www.sciencedaily.com/releases/2005/09/050914090337.htm, accessed 20 March 2008.

Willy, R. W., et al. "Effect of Cessation and Resumption of Static Hamstring Muscle Stretching on Joint Range of Motion." *Journal of Orthopaedic & Sports Physical Therapy* 31(3): 138–144 (2001).

Wright, Vonda J. "Osteoporosis in Men." *Journal of the American Academy of Orthopaedic Surgeons* 14(6): 347–353 (2006).

Wright, Vonda J.; and Perricelli, Brett C. "Age-Related Rates of Decline in Performance Among Elite Senior Athletes." *American Journal of Sports Medicine* 36(3): 443–450 (2008).

Zhao, Emily; Tranovich, Michael J.; and Wright, Vonda J. "The Role of Mobility as a Protective Factor on Cognitive Functioning in Aging Adults: A Review." *Sports Health* 6(1):63–69 (2014).

INDEX

ABOUT THE AUTHORS

VONDA WRIGHT

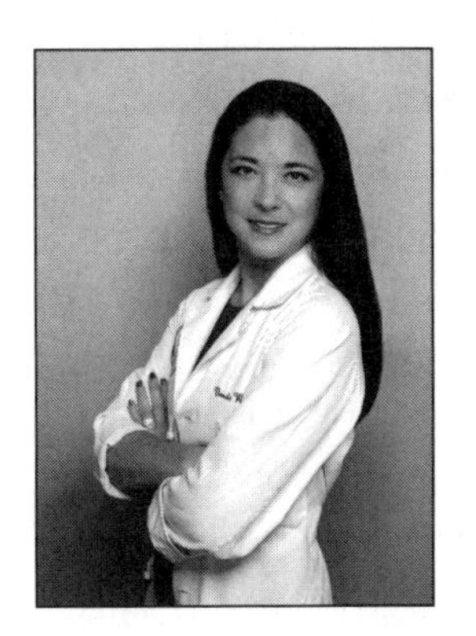

Dr. Vonda Wright is an orthopaedic surgeon, speaker, author, and internationally recognized authority on active aging and mobility. She specializes in sports medicine and is one of only a few female orthopaedic surgeons in the United States. Dr. Wright is the founding director of the Performance and Research Initiative for Masters Athletes (PRIMA) and was recently appointed as the inaugural Medical Director of the UPMC Lemieux Sports Complex. Her pioneering research in mobility and musculoskeletal aging is changing the way we view and treat the aging process.

In addition to performing her surgical practice, Dr. Wright regularly appears on national TV shows, including *The Dr. Oz Show*, *The Doctors*, and *ABC News*. She is frequently quoted in the *Wall Street Journal, New York Times, USA Today*, and *U.S. News & World Report*; in magazines such as *Maxim, Prevention, Fitness, More, Runner's World, Best Life*, and *Arthritis Today*; and in numerous online publications. Dr. Wright speaks worldwide and has authored two mainstream books, *Fitness After 40: How to Stay Strong at Any Age* (the first edition of this book) and *Guide to Thrive: Four Steps to Body, Brains, and Bliss*.

In 2013, Dr. Wright ignited a national conversation on women's health via her online and live conference series, Women's Health Conversations, focused on educating and empowering smart, savvy women to make the best health decisions for themselves and those they touch. For more information, go to www.womenshealthconversations.com.

Dr. Wright earned her first bachelor's degree (in biology) from Wheaton College and her second bachelor's and a master of science (in oncology nursing) from Rush University. She earned her medical degree from the University of Chicago, completed her residency in orthopaedic surgery at the University of Pittsburgh, and completed her fellowship in sports and shoulder surgery at the Hospital for Special Surgery in New York. She is board certified and holds a subspecialty certification in sports medicine.

Dr. Wright currently practices at the UPMC Lemieux Sports Complex and UPMC Hospitals, serves as the "team doc" for five of the University of Pittsburgh Olympic Sports Teams and the Pittsburgh Ballet Theatre, and lives with her husband and their blended family of six children in Pittsburgh.

Connect with Dr. Wright:

Website: www.drvondawright.com
Facebook: facebook.com/DrVonda
Twitter: @DrVondaWright

RUTH WINTER

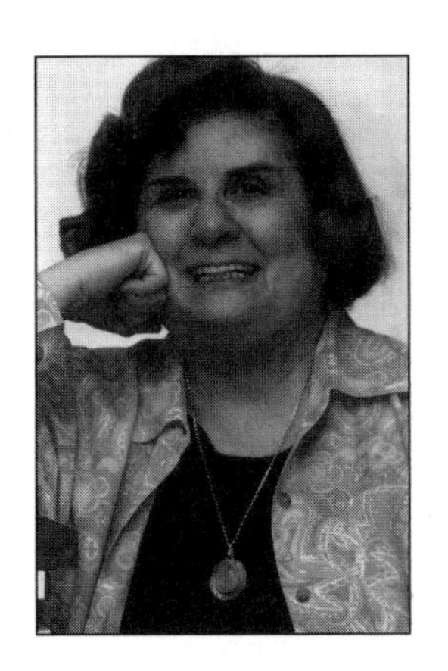

Ruth Winter is an award-winning science writer who has written hundreds of magazine articles and 37 popular health books. She has won many awards including the Career Achievement Award from the American Society of Journalists and Authors (ASJA), the Article Writing Award from the American Medical Writers Association, the Service Award from the National Association of Science Writers, and the Golden Triangle Award from the American Academy of Dermatology. She has published pieces in *Woman's Day, Family Circle,* and *Good Housekeeping*, among other publications. Former science editor of the *Star-Ledger* in New Jersey and nationally syndicated columnist for *The Los Angeles Times*, she specializes in writing about scientific subjects that she makes understandable and interesting to the public. Her late husband, Arthur Winter, M.D., was director of the New Jersey Neurological Institute in Livingston, New Jersey. Ruth Winter has three children, Robin Winter-Sperry, M.D., CEO of Scientific Advantage LLC and its subsidiary MSL Advantage; Craig Winter, a CTO of start-up companies; and Grant Winter, president of realworldtestdrive.com. She also has three grandchildren, Samantha, Hunter, and Katelynd. Her website is ruthwinter.wordpress.com.